Health Essentials

MASSAGE

A practical introduction

STEWART MITCHELL

ELEMENT
Shaftesbury, Dorset • Rockport, Massachusetts
Brisbane, Queensland

© Stewart Mitchell 1992

Published in Great Britain in 1992 by
Element Books Limited
Longmead, Shaftesbury, Dorset

Published in the USA in 1992 by
Element, Inc.
42 Broadway, Rockport, MA 01966

Published in Australia in 1992 by
Element Books Limited for
Jacaranda Wiley Limited
33 Park Road, Milton, Brisbane 4064

Reprinted February 1994

Cover illustration courtesy of Tony Stone Worldwide
Cover design by Max Fairbrother
Typeset by the Electronic Book Factory Ltd, Fife, Scotland
Printed and bound in Great Britain by
Biddles Ltd, Guildford & King's Lynn

British Library Cataloguing in Publication Data
data available

Library of Congress Cataloging in Publication
data available

ISBN 1–85230–386–7

Note from the Publisher

Any information given in any book in the *Health Essentials* series is not intended to be taken as a replacement for medical advice. Any person with a condition requiring medical attention should consult a qualified medical practitioner or suitable therapist.

Contents

Foreword

I have known Stewart Mitchell for ten years as a gifted practitioner and have personal experience of his great skill in massage.

It is good that he also teaches massage, because it is a largely neglected but very effective therapeutic tool. The German word for medical treatment is *behandlung*, which translated literally means 'handling'. This instructive wisdom of language hints at the healing properties of the hands and links up with the 'laying on of hands' in spiritual forms of healing. Stewart has made a careful study of the manifold aspects and benefits of massage – and I am particularly pleased that massage as self-aid and 'mutual help' among family and friends has been investigated as separate from professional massage. In this kind of giving the giver is twice blessed, for we hear so many times that those who massage their friends begin to feel much better themselves.

The chapters are carefully designed so that readers can find at a glance the aspects which are of particular importance to them. I trust that this book will fulfil a real need, and I wish it well!

It is also good to know that Stewart has many years ahead of both teaching and protecting this valuable form of therapy in his friendly and truly nourishing centre in Exeter.

Dr Gordon Latto MB ChB

1

Massage: Its Origins

M ASSAGE IS PERHAPS one of the most popular forms of health activity today. It is effectively used in relaxation groups and workshops, in leisure centres, and as a form of natural therapy. Its origins are both historical and personal.

The art of massage has been practised since ancient times and continues to hold deep significance both for the receiver and the giver; massage offers the experience of touch, movement and energy, qualities associated with the well-being of the whole person.

A word for massage exists in all cultures we have known, and from studies of the classics, it would appear that the ancient Chinese, Greeks and Romans all practised a form of massage.

In some societies massage has been used socially as an act of hospitality, such as in Hawaii where passive movements called *lomi-lomi* are bestowed on honoured guests. Aesthetically, the ancient Greeks associated physical culture with the unfolding of mental and spiritual faculties and set up massage schools in their *gymnasiums*, beautifully built centres of health. In the Far East, performing musicians and actors learn massage practices to aid their artistic development, while exponents of *kathakali*, an early dance form originating in South India, are treated with deep massage from the feet of their teachers.

Working with limited concepts of body-functioning, early physicians were able to use massage effectively in treating fatigue, illness and injury. Hippocrates describes *anatripsis*, literally 'rubbing up', as having a more favourable effect than

1

rubbing down in the limbs, although the understanding of the blood's circulation was at that time incomplete.

It is thought that the development of massage was interrupted with the disintegration of the Greek and Roman civilizations, although an unbroken tradition continued in the East. Not until the sixteenth century and the emergence of relatively sophisticated surgical techniques in France, do we hear of massage re-emerging in Europe in connection with healing.

In the late nineteenth century the demand for therapeutic massage brought about the formation of societies of therapists, with the objects of organizing training, promoting the science of massage and 'safeguarding the interests of the public and the profession'. It is interesting to note the personal requisites for a suitable practitioner of that time:

> Health; not necessarily robust, for often very strong people lack the delicate, empathetic touch required; however, a delicate suffering person cannot expect to do much good to another suffering piece of humanity;

> Intelligence and aptitude; for massage is not so easily done as some might imagine, especially in its adaption to individual cases;

> A high moral tone must be kept at all costs, as much harm has been done by such as do not possess the requisite balance of mind.
>
> Incorporated Society of Massage 1894

The popularity of massage in contemporary times may be explained by a return to 'natural' values in recognition of the highly stressful conditions of modern life. The reaction against unacceptably dehumanizing elements in healthcare in particular has encouraged the revival of therapies which had been discarded in the scientific age.

However, enthusiasm for massage still meets with resistance today. Massage has been abused socially and there can be confusion about it's place in healing; there remains, too, ignorance and misunderstanding of the body.

In the first part of the book and as a thread running through it, reference is made to our wonderful anatomy, with an appeal to the *imagination*, because first of all, anatomy *is* imagination.

Little is meaningfully learned about the body, unless we can imagine, for example, our heart's silent yet powerful beating, the delicacy and strength of muscles and the balance of the bony arrangements which support us.

Massage is a very sensitive and sensitizing form of human contact, whose medium is touch, a sense to which human beings are especially responsive. Among the animals we have one of the longest infancies, during which time we are dependent on safe handling for protection and guidance in the world around us.

The experience of massage could be said to begin from birth, as the muscles of the uterus deliver the baby along the birth canal by rhythmic contraction. After we are born, holding, rocking, washing and caressing by the parent prepares our body for its independence.

As we become more self-controlled, the body's own massage movements become stronger; the movements of our arms and legs against the earth, for example, get us around but are also necessary to help our blood circulate effectively; and the gradual co-ordination of our hands enables us to squeeze and scratch and soothe ourselves from discomfort.

Emotionally, too, as the early Greeks suspected, the quality of our physical contact with the world is very stimulating. While in the womb, we are well protected and our senses are assumed to be dormant; after birth, while we are acquiring knowledge about sounds, focusing our gaze and recognizing smells, we are particularly dependent on the reassurance of touch. Modern research has indicated that given the choice between food and comforting touch *with no food*, the infant is more likely to choose touch.

Thus our connection with the origins of massage can be appreciated as much more immediately personal than a historical perspective suggests; the movements of external, given massage are powerful reminders of the security of touch for the adult.

It should come as no surprise therefore, that those who take up massage find that they have a natural aptitude for it. Massaging is an activity in which it is coaching rather than teaching that is called for. You may be cautious about attending courses introducing the principles of massage, which often range from the basic to the esoteric, but their usefulness is to bring you into contact with others and extend your experience. A good course is one in which you feel *safe*.

A story concerning the Emperor Hadrian (d. AD138) records the origins of the 'massage workshop':

> One day, seeing a soldier easing his back against the marble at the public baths, the Emperor stopped him and inquired why he did so. When the veteran answered that he had no one to massage him, the Emperor, pitying his condition, gave him two attendants and their keep.
>
> The next day when Hadrian appeared again at the baths, a number of citizens began to rub themselves against the wall, hoping to have similar good fortune but the Emperor, divining their intentions, directed them to rub one another!
>
> Copestake, *The Theory and Practice of Massage*,
> Lewis & Co, 1926.

While supporting you to become an original practitioner of massage, this book does not discourage formal massage between professional and client; in fact I recommend that you take advantage of and support professional practices which may be available to you. I'm sure you will find that contact with a therapist becomes increasingly helpful as your own massage skills evolve.

2

Massage for Pleasure, Exercise and Health

O UR EXPERIENCE OF HEALTH helps us to be happy, energetic and purposeful. We may be encouraged to increase our health through personal effort, by following athletic and creative pursuits, or by modifying our behaviours which are deemed to be harmful. A contrasting approach is that health is not a state which can be achieved but an attitude towards life, not struggling for what is already ours.

'Are health and fitness the same?' is a reasonable question, often discussed (at the bar) in leisure centres. The frenetic pursuit of health can be confused with the fear of illness, and guilt from all our 'un-healthy' habits. Asking for a definition of 'health' at a beginners massage group brought varying responses: 'curiosity', 'two evacuations a day', 'no pain', 'freedom from conflict'. There was general agreement that well-intentioned health campaigns can be confusing – for example butter vs. margarine, to jog or not to jog, to keep calm/express emotion.

'Medically fit' was a concept rejected by the group as a minimal definition, which tended to reduce a person to the sum of the body's parts. The idea of a 'body-mind' health emerged and our psychological experience of being *embodied* was discussed. After some lively debate we agreed on a working model: that each body has a 'mind of its own' which is capable of infinite expression – individually, sensually, imaginatively and socially.

For some, health may be related to achievement of personal goals, yet many outstanding athletes and artists have not possessed perfect health; high achievers often speak of the

5

emotional strain of success and the pressures which accompany such individuality. At the other extreme, advice to conform to safe, restrictive practices in the way we eat, drink and proceed in life is not universally convincing – it is rarely disputed that too much dietary fat damages blood vessels, that smoking irritates the lungs or that constant worrying depletes nerves, but avoidance of these behaviours does not appear to *insure* against ill-health.

Are there individual qualities of health which manage to retain an integrated body-mind – in success and failure, in occasional excess, in conserving ourselves and yet having the capacity to 'enjoy' health?

Perhaps we can be inspired by those who, towards the end of their lives, say why they feel so *satisfied*. Not infrequently we hear of their inquisitiveness, their enthusiasm to take risks and become involved in life, without any apparent confidence.

In this book we are going to begin, perhaps tentatively, an appreciation of health, by observing, investigating and experimenting with massage. Take a moment to realize that this will be a serious adventure, in that it could bring you some direct, tangible benefits; at the same time, it's likely to be a truly pleasurable experience!

MOVEMENT

Movement is often regarded as a sign of life; it is certainly an indication of health. This is true not only of speed or strength but especially in co-ordination, since a well co-ordinated body usually feels as good as it looks.

Most of our routine physical tasks are unconsciously directed, yet all were patiently learned. Seemingly effortless movements, however, can revert to clumsiness as soon as we become tired or nervous. How often do we miss the last step or trip on the first and experience a real shock! We don't congratulate ourselves on achieving simple tasks and yet we are indignant when we fail; we take the skill of our movement for granted, including the satisfaction that it gives. We only fully appreciate our mobility when we lose it and perhaps for this reason someone who develops a 'bad back' or a stiff neck can be difficult to live with.

Some of our most complicated movements take place inside the body, strictly unconscious and beyond our voluntary control: the circulation of the blood, propulsion of food through the intestines, and erection of body hairs for example. Curiously, these movements are accomplished equally effectively by the lazy as they are by the fit. This is because the effort comes from what we are made up of as well as what we do with ourselves. It can explain why some people appear to maintain their health in spite of their habits rather than by trying to be healthy.

The oft-quoted 'fifty-cigarettes-a-day-bottle-of-scotch-TV-addict' (who lived until he was eighty years old) is invariably dead by the time we hear about him but we could consider that even health abuse can have an athletic quality to it. What is worth noting is that the more fixed and mundane the motivation of the health seeker, the less real movement is taking place if health becomes a goal in itself.

Our body's mechanical dimension can be seen on the outside but few of us are on truly intimate terms with our interiors and even our back is 'behind' us. For children, having a body is exciting – it's new! Our early activities are full of surprises; even our mistakes such as dropping things and falling over are fun, and we don't feel the pain or embarrassment this can cause us as adults. In adulthood we are tenser and have much more to lose from our errors. We pay the price for this tension with a diminished sense of fun.

For an exercise (Figure 1), try crawling around the room on all fours like you once did, or see how long you can stand on one leg. How do you feel doing this? Uncomfortable, afraid, or do you get a sneaking sense of relief from the strain of being grown-up?

HANDS

Take a good look at your hands and move them gently. In spite of any personal reservations you might have, from the point of view of structure, sensitivity and aesthetics, your hands are unsurpassed. They contain the ability to perform incredible tasks. Interestingly, you may have noticed that

7

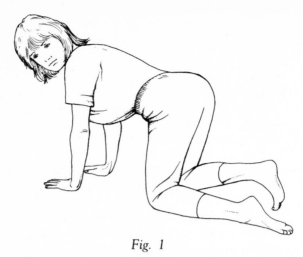

Fig. 1

there are few muscles in the hand: wriggle your fingers while watching your forearms, and you will notice your finger bones are operated from a distance by arm muscles, like puppetry. Otherwise the constant movement of muscular hands would make them grow too big for their delicate manipulations.

Are you equally familiar with both hands? How many bones can you count in your fingers ? How do you explain that your hand can turn a door handle without your body doing a cartwheel?

Together with all their skills of dexterity, hands have great powers of sense, having amongst the most numerous of nerve endings of any part of the skin. The eyes are dependent on the hands to confirm reality. Our early development of hand–eye co-ordination is very important, and later in life if we are plunged into darkness our hands reliably take over. Asked how they would negotiate a darkened room, people might say by sound or echo or by visualizing previous impressions, but quite probably their hands would immediately be reaching out – recognizing, guiding and solving the problem.

This book presents the opportunity to realize just how much our hands can be relied upon therapeutically. Our hands are there as the tools and the means to encourage our bodies to health.

THE PLEASURE OF MASSAGE

Even if the *idea* of massage might be attractive, enjoyment of a massage is not something that is immediately acceptable to everyone. There are many reasons for this, not least that if you were not handled agreeably as a child, you are unlikely to trust being handled as an adult. Fortunately, the body is designed in such a way as to be constantly massaging itself and this can give us some confidence to begin with:

- the diaphragm muscle between the chest and abdomen alternately compresses and releases the digestive organs with each deep breath;
- even the slightest movement of the limb muscles squeeze and relieve pressure on the nearby veins to keep peripheral circulation flowing;
- the arms, kept free to swing by the sides as we walk, relax the muscles of the back.

If we are able to imagine this, we are on the way to appreciating the advantages offered by applied massage.

Two everyday examples further illustrate the value of massage:

1. When we are unwell or tired, many of our natural body movements become depressed. You may notice that if you have to sit still over a long period of time your lower legs seem to 'fill up'. If you've slipped your shoes off, as you might do on a long journey, they will probably feel harder to put back on. This is because the natural massaging movements of the legs have been inhibited by sitting still, and the effect of gravity is slowing down the extreme circulations. Unremedied, this situation may induce a headache or drowsiness. After a few minutes of simple massage movements, of wringing and stroking, however, the situation can be corrected for the comfort of the whole body.
2. Most of us will have experienced the stiffening, locally or over a larger area of the body, which comes after a collision or fall or even an unpleasant emotional exchange. Muscles and joints which normally glide effortlessly under our skin become painfully reluctant and we assume a cautious posture.

Here, massage intervention can be valuable by not only easing and loosening our condition but also creating a reassuring atmosphere within the body. Perhaps, left to ourselves, we would recover our composure but very often we are too busy or exhausted to complete the job effectively.

INVITATION TO HEALTH

To maintain or recover health it is possible to have 'treatment' or perhaps to 'study' health or read books about it. The exciting and rewarding possibilities of massage are that it offers a combination of these approaches. You will receive benefits both in giving and receiving massage, and may find new perspectives in health. People new to massage often express delight in their rediscovery of touch and movement – as receivers, in their capacity to respond, and in giving, in the heightened awareness of their senses and interpretation.

The material for this book is drawn directly from treatments and classwork which people have found to be useful and enjoyable. In both treating and teaching, I have found the acquisition of specific techniques secondary to the development of sensitivity; consequently, the theme of this book is how the appreciation and enjoyment of health is already in our hands.

3

Moving Experiences: The Anatomy of Movement

OUR INTELLIGENT MUSCLES

OUR BODY IS an accomplished mover. Compared with other creatures, we may not be as elegant, fast or strong but only in the human form are physical attributes combined to such a high degree.

External movements are enacted by muscles consciously working in conjunction with bones, while internally the muscular system is a main promoter of health – by creating heat and stimulating the circulation of blood, digestion and respiratory processes. Even when apparently at rest, the muscles vibrate in anticipation of movement. This enables us to jump into action at extremely short notice, whether to avert danger or to eject a morsel of food which has found its way into our windpipe. A detailed description of the body's structure and function is astonishing.

This introduction to the muscles may encourage you to persevere in your study of movement.

Many massagers find it frustrating to have to integrate an intellectual understanding of the body with their spontaneous and intuitive feelings for massage. This is worth trying to overcome, since the more you massage the more you will want to know what is happening while you are massaging.

Although we have an intimate relationship with our body, how it functions can be mystifying. Unless you have studied the human body in biology lessons, the most common occasion for self-scrutiny is during an illness or injury, not always a positive experience, when the body's workings can be even more misunderstood.

Remembering that our body is something which moves, even when it is represented pressed flat between the pages of a textbook, we can begin to explore anatomy from our general knowledge. The formal language of anatomy need not be intimidating. Terminology is often a concise expression for a familiar image: the word 'muscle' for example is derived from the Latin for 'little mouse' to describe the way the skin ripples when a muscle moves underneath.

Using the cut-out model in the Appendix, it is possible to create a clearer, more vivid anatomy of the moving body. You will also learn a great deal about the body from observing everyday movements, especially those we take for granted. Noticing the different ways we get in and out of cars or catch a falling object is just as relevant to massage as reading about muscle action. There are many excellent books on human anatomy for in-depth study, but to begin with use your own and your friends' bodies experimentally.

The spinal column is the pivotal structure for all movement and, together with our developed buttock muscles, distinguishes our posture from that of other creatures. Curiously, we have come to regard our buttocks as 'seats' when in fact these muscles are primarily responsible for our ability to stand upright for long periods. This is in contrast to a kangaroo, for example, which needs a long flat tail for upright balance, and even the apes are obliged to drop down on to their knuckles occasionally; we have the freedom to use our upper limbs for more sophisticated purposes – like massage!

The muscles of our lower back are not easily strained, in spite of the great tensions which can accumulate there, unless we lift ourselves (and sometimes even the lightest object) awkwardly. We are then aware of our back 'going', which is more likely to be a muscular response than the infamous disc which does not actually 'slip'. Human evolution is then temporarily reversed and we react by dropping forward on to our hands so as to take the weight of the body from the spine; relief usually comes from lying as flat as possible.

Dramatic as these incidents can be, the spine is actually much more vulnerable to habitual postures which unbalance its tensions. Although we are accustomed to referring to the

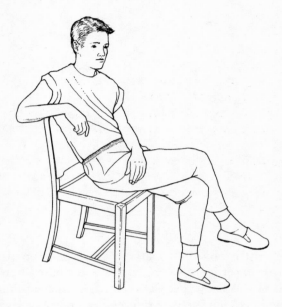

Fig. 2

spine as the 'back' its position is closer to the centre of the
body, and almost all the postural muscles are attached to it.
While one end of the column may be under stress from the
legs, the other end has to maintain the poise of the head –
a truly remarkable achievement. As long as the alignment is
maintained there is almost no limit to the spine's continual
performance. The Western tendency to cross the legs (thighs)
when seated, however, is very undermining for the spine
(Figures 2 and 3).

   We usually have a preference for one leg over the other,
which creates a constant twisting and shortening of the deep
pelvic muscles. One way of observing the impact of habitually
sitting this way is to observe the symmetry of your partner's
legs when they lie down before a treatment. Not unusually,
one foot will lie more upright than the other which falls away
with the more relaxed leg to the outside. Looking more closely
at the pelvis, you may observe that the ileum bone (where the

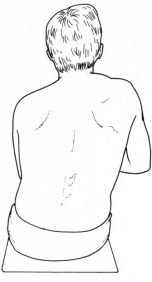

Fig. 3

hands go on the hips) is relatively prominent on the same side as the tenser leg; this confirms the increased tension on one side of the body. People affected in this way may also experience neckache to one side by the end of a day and, if female, increased pressure at one side of the abdomen during menstruation.

Your massages will have reduced influences if your partner is a confirmed 'leg-crosser'. We cross the legs for many apparently helpful reasons – to rest a book on, to combat feelings of self-consciousness, or because it seems a sophisticated way to sit. Only when we begin to feel it is not so advantageous (our leg goes numb) are we inclined to uncross. This urgent, conscious sensation is really merely an indication of far-reaching strains occurring throughout our spine's posture.

Often accompanying leg-crossing, and potentially as strenuous, is forward projection of the head when concentrating either at a desk or in a car (Figure 4). Tension in the neck spine goes unrelieved until we get really tired, by which time the neck muscles will have become rigid.

The neck has seven separate bones, which together with the head above and the chest below means we have eight joints for potential movement. Neck-rolling exercises are not ideal

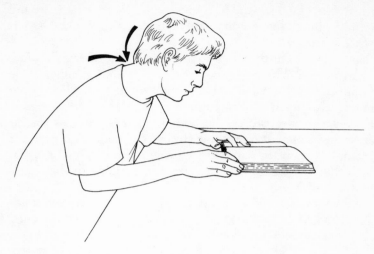

Fig. 4

for these joints especially if the tensions have become focused at one joint.

Both the lower back and the neck are great centres of nervous control in the body and therefore very sensitive to conditions of strain. Fortunately this 'nervousness' also makes for receptivity to massage. Deep strokes around the spinal column can relax or invigorate the deeper and peripheral areas of the body; and when massage is used remedially on any one part, attention is always given to the spine to reinforce the effects of that treatment.

THE CUT OUT MODEL (see pages 117–19)

The Bones

Our bones are known collectively as the skeleton, which means 'dried up'. Contrary to their appearance in the classroom, in life bones are extremely dynamic and versatile structures. They are not only concerned with movement but also provide protection for organs such as the brain, and are involved in the production of blood cells. You are quite likely to know the name of some bones from common knowledge. Notice that the end of the longer forearm bone (ulna) is what we regard as the elbow;

its near neighbour, (radius) is the bone which rotates around it and allows the familiar but complex unscrewing action of the hand.

It is also interesting to compare the pelvis with the shoulder arrangement. The collar bone (clavicle) and shoulder-blade (scapula) are the important structures for arm muscles, whose movements further distinguish us from the other creatures. However, if we divorce the arms from their normal role as an accompaniment to walking (by carrying a heavy object, for example) when they should be swinging in diagonal rhythm with the legs, we soon notice strain developing in the back's postural muscles.

Bones are very light yet extremely strong, and like scaffolding poles can withstand great stress. If a simple fracture occurs, the bone's healing is usually so complete that it is unlikely that it will break again at the same point. General massage of the remainder of the body is beneficial while fractures are immobilized for healing, and very supportive when your partner is regaining the use of a healed bone.

Introduce yourself and your partner to their bones by tracing them on the diagram and under their skin.

The Muscles

Muscles are everywhere in the body, making up the mass of our weight and shape. Some are easy to locate and have individual names like the well-known Biceps, which helps flex the elbow.

The numerous erector muscles of the body hairs are detected only in their effects, as when the hairs stand on end to keep the heat within the skin. Muscles only contract (i.e. shorten) to cause a movement, and rely on the contraction of their opposite neighbouring muscles to relax out.

You can illustrate this for yourself: Straighten your elbow. If both the Biceps (at the front of the upper arm) and the Triceps (at the rear) contract simultaneously, the elbow locks straight; when the Biceps increases its contraction the Triceps agrees to relax and the elbow flexes. Beginning again from this position, try the movement in reverse.

Muscles are wonderfully responsible. They give us strength, help keep the blood warm, cushion us, and reliably guard against collisions with our environment. For example, if we should fall over we would be wise to let the larger muscles take the impact rather than an outstretched hand and risk an arm fracture.

Muscles faithfully record our feelings, and their tensions help ease stressful situations. However, when this tension is not relaxed sufficiently, the lining of the muscles and surrounding tissues are irritated, creating the classic condition known as *fibrositis*. Almost everyone has had this experience of tension, and massage is justly famous for alleviating it.

Even when you might think that you are sitting quite still, all your muscles continue to twitch at a very low level which enables you to spring into action at short notice. Someone has been officially recorded as appearing to be standing completely still for more than twenty-four hours, but a short experiment on your part will demonstrate that your muscles resent under-use even more than over-use.

Assembling the Model

Returning now to the cut-out model, the muscles should be cut out and laid on to the skeleton according to the lowest number first. This corresponds to the way they are arranged on the body, so try to follow the form of your partner's body at the same time.

Begin again with muscle 1 and stick point O with its bony end to the skeleton, leaving the remainder of the muscle to flap. This represents how the muscle is anchored to one bone while its other end inserts (point I) into another bone which it will move. Gradually complete the model according to the instructions in the Appendix on p.116, identifying the actual muscle on your partner as you proceed. The names of the bones and muscles may seem cumbersome compared to the Anglo-Saxon words we are accustomed to but they allow us to enter into the international language of anatomy.

Understanding the body from its basic structures will contribute to your sensitivity towards it and may enable you to help your massage partners with deeper and persistent tensions. Together, you will dispel some of the myths created by experts whose reliance on terminology has tended to make health sound like a secret.

4

How We Massage

TURNING OUR HANDS TO HEALTH

A LTHOUGH MASSAGERS TEND to become concentrated in their hands, even after a little experience you will begin to appreciate that giving massage involves your whole body: your back muscles hold you poised and accommodate the weight of your partner; your legs transfer your weight and give depth to the treatment; the upper arms provide the strength for your strokes. It is in the forearm and hand, however, that the exceptionally detailed manipulations of massage are produced.

Your aim is to be as relaxed as your partner while giving massage, otherwise your tension may become contagious. To avoid tension and the occupational strains associated with giving massage, consider these aspects of your own anatomy.

The Back

Arm and leg muscles tire. more easily than those of the back. (Remembering this, you will appreciate how tired your partner's body must be when they present an aching back.) Massagers inadvertently develop their own backaches by a combination of unrelieved bending, dependence on a preferred hand, and a degree of nervousness in treating which inhibits muscular co-ordination.

To avoid your own back aching in the course of a massage, use the effleurage stroke consistently (see p.22), slightly

18

leaning away from your partner. This will stretch out your upper back and, by re-aligning the head with the spine momentarily, lower back pressure is relieved. Occasionally retracting the abdominal muscles and standing as close as you can to the table, with bent knees, will also minimize back strain.

Massagers should regularly employ first aid and other self-treating methods (*see* Chapter 8).

The Legs

Whether you stand or sit to give treatment, the leg muscles are used to give rhythm to your strokes. If your partner is on a couch, stand halfway along, close in, and see if you can comfortably reach their head or feet without moving a step. Bend both knees as you do this and feel how this is also much easier for your back when you are leaning across.

If you still cannot reach the extremities, the table is too high: make a small running board to massage from, rather than sawing down the legs of the couch, in case you end up with a couch that is too low.

When kneeling, use your thigh muscles to lift and lower your hips when reaching across your partner. A massage stool is very useful for kneelers who have stiff ankles or cannot take all their weight on their feet.

The Arms

Pushing and pulling movements are accomplished by muscles which attach the upper arm to the shoulders and chest. To develop your strength exercises like push-ups and pull-ups are sometimes recommended. You may have to do these if you find yourself tiring initially, but regular massaging itself creates strength proportionately.

The design of the lower arm is quite fantastic. Place your arm, palm upward, on a table in front of you: you will see in your forearm many muscles crowding together, passing through the narrowness of your wrist; in the palm of your hand the muscles extend to reach along the fingers. Some of the muscles stop at the palm bones, enabling the hand to be turned in almost any direction, like an 'angle-poise'. The study of the lower arm is one of the most difficult in anatomy but it is also aesthetically very pleasing.

The Hands

It is peculiar to observe that when curling the fingers, the arm muscles begin twitching, although this actually happens the other way around. Turn your arm over to see a corresponding arrangement for opening the hand and stretching the fingers. Our hands can therefore remain slender but very strong, and the many joints in the fingers give almost limitless dexterity. There is nothing in all of nature to compare with the engineering of our hands.

While the skin over our palms is relatively thick, it contains massive numbers of nerve endings, second only to the feet, for heightened sensitivity. Our fingers can be relied on as much as our eyes, as this massager's game illustrates:

Sit with a partner. The first person draws a simple design (say, three dots) with a fingertip on the other's palm, while the partner closes their eyes. Then, with eyes open, the partner attempts to construct the design on the first person's palm.

If the reconstruction is accurate, the first person repeats and adds a little more design to the partner's palm. See how complicated you can make the design, and then swap roles when your partner cannot complete a design.

You will be surprised to find how successful you can become at following your partner's design with your sense of touch rather than your eyes. Progress in massage is related to how much we are able to respond to information received in our hands, and this game is useful for beginners and as a refresher for experienced practitioners.

STROKES

The many different strokes of massage were rationalized by a Swede, Professor Henry Ling in the nineteenth century. His 'Swedish System' was incorporated into medicine but its reputation has suffered both in the popular image of the massage 'parlour' and in its declining use in physiotherapy, which has become more mechanized.

This is an unfortunate association for Ling's original work, which is very relevant for all massagers. Ling was the first Westerner to give a physiology of massage, showing the direct physical and psychological benefits of particular movements. Visualizing these effects as we work is helpful, especially in our early days of practice when self-confidence is important. Having an image of the stroke tends to dispel the tension which can develop in your hands if you are trying too hard, and your partner may also appreciate your ability to explain what you are doing, confirming that the good experience they are having is indeed beneficial.

Experiencing the different strokes

As a 'warm-up' before giving massage, you might like to use these suppling and strengthening exercises:

1. Widen your elbows and place your fingertips together; press slowly until each finger is stretched flat against its opposite, wrists fully flexed. Lower the hands to increase the stretch.

2. Make fists, then throw out the fingers as wide apart and as straight as possible; hold for ten seconds and repeat six times.

3. Relax your hands and shake vigorously from the wrists in all directions, keeping your elbows flexed and your arms still. Stop when your hands feel 'rubbery' and your fingers tingle.

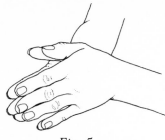

Fig. 5

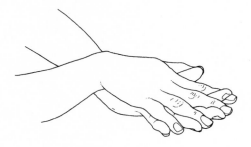

Fig. 6

Try the next exercise slowly as it is very demanding on the hands and wrists:

4. (a) Put your hands flat against each other (Figure 5); cross them right over left and interlock the fingers (Figure 6).
(b) Let your elbows widen and open at your hands while keeping your fingers interlocked (Figures 7 and 8).
(c) Drop both elbows and extend both arms, right above left, until the palms face forward . . . but with fingers still interlocked (Figure 9). Repeat, beginning with hands crossed left over right.

This exercise is initially achieved by only ten per cent of students, not just because it is difficult but also very confusing! Persevere, as it is the supreme movement for relieving stiffness and tiredness in the hands and forearms.

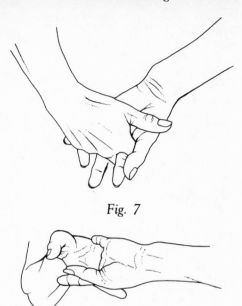

Fig. 7

Fig. 8

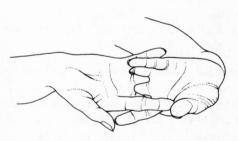

Fig. 9

Ling's classical strokes define massage as a combination of three movements, *effleurage*, *petrissage*, and *percussion* (use your own body or your massage partner's to experience how they are done and how they feel):

1. Slowly stroke an expanse of skin, say on the forearm or thigh, using the whole surface of the palm of your hand,

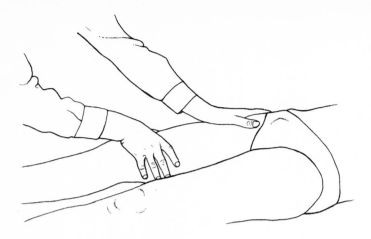

Fig. 10

fingers relaxed (Figure 10). This is *effleurage*, the preparatory and background stroke. You will feel that this is soothing, while gently bringing your attention to the part which is being touched. Effleurage is 'non-invasive' since it puts no pressure into the body and does not attempt to move it; this is very important at the beginning and end of a massage. Although superficial in comparison with other strokes, effleurage is profound in its effects due to the skin's nervous connections with deeper parts of the body.

- *Effleurage stroke enables you to attune with your partner, while planning and reviewing your treatment.*
- *Effleurage is appreciated by slender or anxious partners.*
- *Effleurage is a good discipline in patience for massagers who can't wait to 'get on with the massage'!*

2a. Take hold of an edge of the body (for example, the inside thigh) with your fingertips. Move along making squeezing strokes using the balls of your thumbs – this is *petrissage* (Figure 11). This type of pressure is suitable on sinewy muscles found in the limbs and upper back. Petrissage adjusts their tension rather than forcing it out, which they would resist. (If the forearm muscles are squeezed too hard, for example, the fingers will contract involuntarily.)

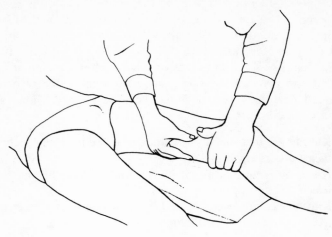

Fig. 11

- Petrissage stroke allows detailed work on the body.
- Petrissage is recommended on children and older adults.
- Petrissage develops sensitivity in the fingers.

2b. Most people associate massage with the deep stroke, *kneading*, where curved muscles, such as those on the front of the thigh are squeezed with the whole hand and thumb (Figure 12). This stroke is used to break down deep tensions and condition muscles to have even tension. Encouraging the muscles to be

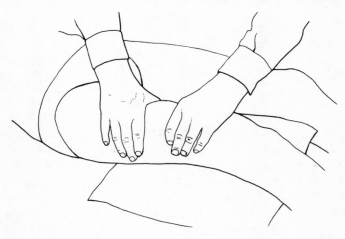

Fig. 12

25

more sponge-like helps local circulation and assists the heart; kneading also seems to convey to a partner that 'something is being done' about their condition! Depending on the shape of a large muscle, kneading can also be done with the heel of the hand or foot, knuckles or elbow. However, groans of delight can give way to tears, since the experience of being kneaded can be very emotional because deep tensions are being released.

- *Kneading is best suited for partners who are muscular and use their muscles vigorously.*
- *Kneading requires strength in the arms and thumb muscles, which will develop with practice.*
- *Kneading can be overdone and both massager and partner will feel tired – interrupt with effleurage.*

3. So that those receiving massage can pick themselves up, feeling relaxed but also ready to face life again, a massage is completed by skilful striking of the body. Ling calls this stroke *percussion*, using wrist movement to stimulate the body with different parts of the hand. Percussion is designed to reintegrate the muscles, lessening the contrast from deep relaxation back into everyday movement.

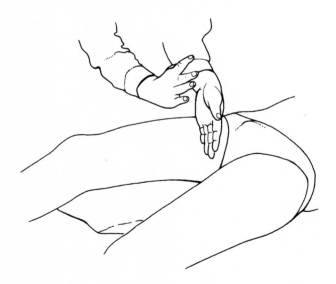

Fig. 13

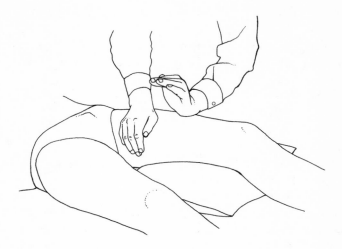

Fig. 14

Hacking is a general percussion, done lightly with the fingers (as seen in popular representations of massage): parallel your palms, fingers slightly stretched and chop from the wrist so that the lower three fingers make contact with the body, while vibrating against each other (Figure 13). Hack slowly, then build up speed and depth.

- *Hacking causes muscles to 'wake up' without disturbing your partner's sense of relaxation.*

Cupping is used on the lower back and can be helpful over the rib case: make your hands into a 'cup' that would be watertight; turn upside down and beat the body by alternately flexing the wrists (Figure 14). Begin slowly, maintaining the cup as you increase in speed and depth. You will hear a hollow sound as the air is beaten from the surface of the skin; finger marks on the skin reveal that the cup is too shallow and your partner will be feeling the percussion uncomfortably.

- *Cupping encourages deep circulation in the large muscles and prepares them for action.*

27

Tapotement is the lightest percussion, mostly applied around the face and head and to sensitive or injured areas: drum your fingertips across the face avoiding direct contact with the eyes. On larger areas the fingers are kept together and tapped against the skin.

● *Tapotement, when used monotonously, becomes very soothing and can be used to numb aching muscles or irritated skin.*

Ling's system describes a formula for strokes which offer a satisfactory massage:

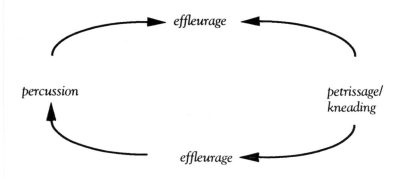

Effleurage is the introductory and concluding stroke as well as the background to all other strokes; rather than pause between strokes, apply effleurage as you review your treatment plan to give a soothing continuity to the massage.

Petrissage and kneading release hypertensions in the body and distribute the muscles evenly around the skeleton. Temporarily holding their body firmly relieves the onus on our partner to manage their own tension, (hence the oft-heard appeal: 'Don't stop!'); our movements become an auxiliary muscle system for their body.

Percussions, coming at the end of treatment, introduce a helpful mini-tension to partners to prepare them for renewed activity. Lightly striking the muscles will 'immunize' them against greater pressure in everyday life and should not feel like a punishment!

I recommend that you begin your practice on the basics of the Swedish System to gain the trust of your partner; you will be able to explain clearly *what* you are doing and *why*. Your own particular style will develop from the interpretation you give to the strokes and the reactions they produce. Don't feel that you have to 'get it right' according to Ling's formula, which is intended only as a initial guide but do make sure you check with your partner that your enthusiasm is being matched by their appreciation.

'TALKING HANDS'

While it is good to have explanations for your work, verbal conversation can often interrupt the feedback from touch. In silence, new sensations arising into consciousness can intercept tensions and allow the benefits of the treatment to last longer. You are certainly not obliged to give a running commentary on your massage and you may occasionally feel that you want to discourage too much questioning from a nervous partner. Changes in tension can bring up feelings of insecurity, however, and although with practice you should be able to anticipate this, be ready to respond verbally if your partner needs reassurance.

During massage our hands hold a conversation with our partner's muscles. We can ask for postures and movements which may or may not depend on our partner's conscious understanding.

Exercise

Compare the influence of verbal communication with that of your hands alone for remedying this everyday shoulder tension:

Have your partner sitting down on a couch and stand directly behind them. You will observe that one shoulder is held higher than the other, often in association with the preferred hand.

Request that they shrug their shoulders and release, especially on the raised side. Usually, partners are unsuccessful in relaxing the higher shoulder. If so, try this:

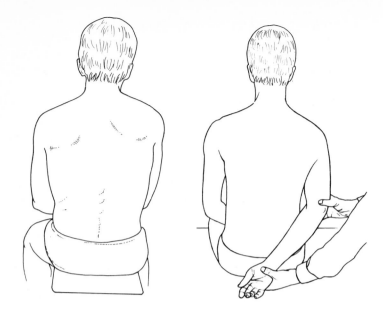

Fig. 15   Fig. 16

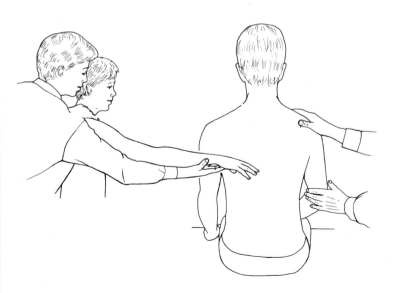

Fig. 17   Fig. 18

Place your partner's hands into their lap (Figure 15). Gently lift the arm on the tense side and fold it behind their back (Figure 16). Let the arm hang and lightly stroke it from the shoulder to the elbow.

Support the whole weight of the arm and lift it up and around to the front of the body, then extend it straight out in front (Figure 17).

Lower the arm slowly and replace it into the lap (Figure 18).

Stand back and look again at the shoulders; the tense side will now be *lower* than the other. Make the same movements with the other arm to even up the shoulders.

If your massage practice is becoming too routine or you are not feeling satisfied with your strokes, you may simply be tired, so don't forget to have an occasional massage yourself! Re-reading this chapter might also help you to become more aware of how your massage is progressing and will remind you of the intended effects of the strokes. Remember that relaxation, poise and awareness in your hands is generally appreciated by partners more than too much effort.

5

Practical Massage

EVERYDAY MASSAGES FOR EACH PART OF THE BODY

Setting

M ASSAGES ARE GIVEN in whichever situation seems appropriate. Most professionals have a quiet room and a treatment couch but you might like to use a kitchen table or chair, and some massagers find the floor perfectly suitable. It is important that both people involved are equally comfortable with the atmosphere of the situation.

Whether you use talc or oil with your massage depends on style as well as your partner's preference. Talc can be useful at the beginning of massage, while oil is helpful in detailed work. Anxiety at the early stage of treatment can cause both people to sweat, which makes effleurage difficult, and massage strokes on very dry skin can create uncomfortable friction. Thus you may like to use talc for convenience early in the treatment or for the first massage. Oil massage can be recommended for children and older adults because it deflects too much direct pressure away from the body. Massage to loosen a stiff or painful joint can also be a suitable occasion for utilizing the gliding influence of oil. Add oil a little at a time on to your hand first, rather than direct to the body.

I recommend that you practise using neither of these lubricants. Direct contract between your hand and your partner's skin is necessary in recognizing tension and the condition of muscles. Not everyone necessarily wants to be rubbed with an oily or powdery substance just to experience massage, but some people definitely do when it helps them to relax; you will easily find out.

Most adults approach their first massage with a variety of preconceptions. Regardless of your approach, your partner may expect massage to be an athletic or hedonistic experience, be both threatening and relaxing, daringly sexual, or completely clinical. The actual massage will soon clarify these thoughts, for what is really at issue for your partner is how they are used to being 'handled', both at present and when they were very young.

This psychological aspect means that partners are particularly vulnerable to the first and last touch of massage; make sure that the beginning and ending of your treatments are slow and gentle, careful and reassuring.

A body massage is not necessarily given in any special order but you might like to follow the sequence in this chapter for practice. For someone new to the treatment, hand massage (see p. 34) can be a good way to begin as it provides a familiar point of contact and you can look at and talk to each other in the usual way.

When not to massage

You should always make some enquiries about your partner's general health before giving massage. When massage is given for the purpose of relaxation and support, it is very unlikely that someone's medical condition will disqualify them from receiving it. However, if any of the conditions below apply to your partner, keep the strokes well within their comfort.

You will be fortunate to find someone who has never been on the checklist. When you are massaging by mutual consent, either person can sense when something does not feel right; if this happens, discontinue and discuss. Your own fitness is relevant too. Your partner may want a vigorous or calming massage, whether you have the capacity on that day or not. What actually occurs in a treatment is the responsibility of both people. In this sharing sense, if any of the checks apply to the receiver or giver of massage, then go gently.

Has your partner recently:

Taken regular medication?
Undergone surgery?
Had an accident or injury?
Undergone osteopathic or chiropractice treatment?
Is your partner pregnant or menstruating?

Although there are serious states of health in which massage is contra-indicated, it is very likely that massage is being denied to more people whose condition would benefit from treatment than could ever be harmed by it. When you are unsure about someone's suitability for treatment, consult an experienced practitioner.

Massage of the Hand

The hand is a natural introduction to the rest of the body with its many muscles, joints and varying thickness of skin. Apart from local soothing benefits, massaging the hands reduces pressure in the neck and head by nervous and circulatory effects.

1. Have your partner lie down with their right arm flexed and resting on the elbow, with a small pillow underneath.
2. Effleurage the hand between your hands, softly squeezing down from the fingertips to the wrist, like a glove being pulled on (Figure 19). Move back to the fingertips with a lighter pressure and repeat 12–20 times.
3. Petrissage by turning the palm downwards, placing your fingertips and thumbs on to the back of the hand, and squeeze all over. Stroke the back of the hand with your thumbs 12 times.
4. Turn the hand upwards and squeeze the palm and base of the thumb.
5. Effleurage as at 2., firmly upwards.
6. Support the hand and percuss it lightly all over with your stiffened fingers.
7. Effleurage lightly.

    Place your partner's hand on to their abdomen, then treat the other hand.

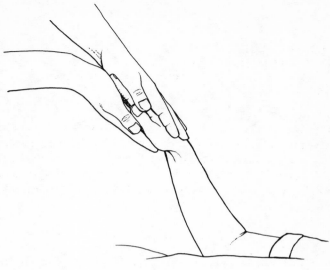

Fig. 19

Congratulations if this is your first massage! Ask your partner for comments and criticisms and tell them anything interesting you noticed about their hands. Later you may prefer to let your treatments speak for themselves.

'Breathing Body' Sequence

A general massage beginning with the back of the trunk is very effective in quickly relaxing the postural muscles. Conveniently, some partners find it easier to settle into a treatment by not facing the massager.

As an introduction to the back you might like to use this 'Breathing Body' sequence. It creates a calm atmosphere and gives you an opportunity to observe something very subtle about the skeleton:

1. Have your partner lie face down. Place a pillow under the abdomen and feet. The arms can be placed around the head or by the sides (Figure 20).
2. Place one hand lightly on the middle of the back and the other over the pelvis. Invite your partner to relax and breathe deeply. You will notice the rise and fall of

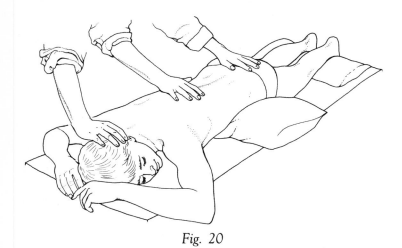

Fig. 20

the chest with breathing – can you feel a corresponding, though softer, movement at the pelvis?

3. Remove your hand from the back and place it lightly on the back of the skull. After a few moments the pelvic movement will become more obvious.
4. Now concentrate on the skull to detect a fainter movement.

Orthodox anatomy teaches that hardly any movement occurs in a stationary pelvis and none at all in the skull; with practice you will become aware that all three areas do actually move in harmony with the breathing. By the time you have completed the sequence, both you and your partner will feel composed and ready to continue the treatment.

Massage of the Back

The complete back massage usually takes 15–20 minutes, certainly not much longer if a whole body treatment is being given.

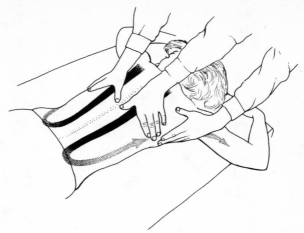

Fig. 21

1. Take up position at your partner's head, facing down the length of the body.
2. Effleurage by gliding softly down the centre of the back with both hands and return via the edges of the body, up to the arms (Figure 21). Repeat 10 times, increasing in depth.
3. Knead using the heels of the hands and the palms to press diagonally across the whole back, up and down, for 30 seconds (Figure 22). Repeat effleurage 5 times.
4. Move to the side of your partner. Lean over and effleurage

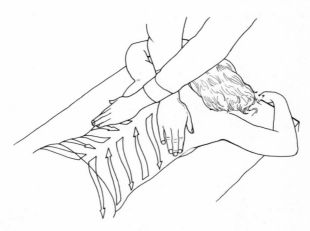

Fig. 22

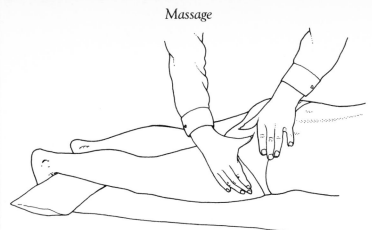

Fig. 23

the opposite buttock. Knead for 30 seconds (Figure 23). Effleurage deeply in a circular motion. Do percussion (cupping) on the buttock for 10 seconds. Effleurage lightly.

5. Effleurage the edge of the chest. Do petrissage from the armpit to the waist and back again for 30 seconds (Figure 24). Effleurage deeply towards the armpit. Do percussion (hacking) for 10 seconds. Effleurage lightly.
6. Effleurage the top of the shoulder from head to arm. Do petrissage for 30 seconds (Figure 25). Do percussion (hacking) for 10 seconds. Effleurage in a circular motion.
7. Walk round to the other side of the body, keeping your hand in contact with the body and repeat all the strokes.
8. Return to position 1. Effleurage as before, this time getting lighter and slower towards the 10th stroke.

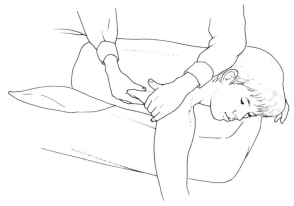

Fig. 24

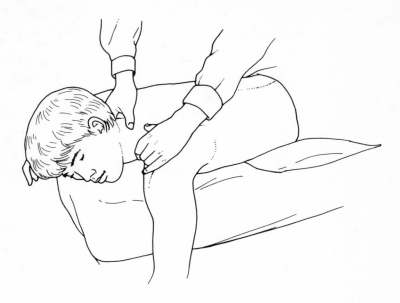

Fig. 25

9. Cover the back with a towel and ask your partner to breathe deeply 3 times.

How is *your* back after giving back massage? This is potentially the most strenuous of treatments, and very tense partners make an unyielding surface to work on. You must be aware of how much bending is involved to reach all parts of the back and make use of the respite of effleurage when you get tired. Remember to keep your knees slightly flexed and don't be tempted to spend more than 20 minutes on back massage.

Ask your partner to turn over slowly. Otherwise they may make make an awkward movement if drowsy, or leap up too fast – and off the couch. Position yourself close to guard against this but don't attempt to lift your partner: instead, develop expertise in removing the pillows from underneath and have them ready to go under the head and thighs as your partner lies

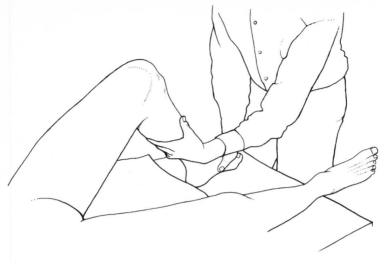

Fig. 26

back. The pillows are important to enable a partner to relax their limbs and neck and will also prolong the effects of the back massage.

Leg Massage

Extraordinary balancers and locomotors, the leg muscles are also adept massagers of their own veins, redirecting spent blood back to the heart against considerable force of gravity. Cardiac patients, formerly ordered to bed and told not to move are now advised to make active leg movements to relieve the strain on their hearts. Commonplace symptoms of cramp and varicosity indicate tiredness in the legs and too much tension above them – treat the legs!

1. Take up position at the feet, facing your partner. Massage the foot of the nearest leg in the same manner as the hand, although all strokes can be deeper unless your partner is very sensitive. After squeezing around the big toe, knead down the instep and back again 6 times.
2. Bend the leg and stand the foot flat. (If your partner suffers varicosity omit the kneading and percussion strokes.)
3. Effleurage with your palm and fingers taking the shape

of the lower leg (Figure 26). Stroke from the ankle to the knee, increasing depth, with a stronger up stroke. Do 20 times.

4. Knead by squeezing and rolling the calf muscles and press against the outside of the shin with your thumb for 30 seconds. Effleurage deeply 5 times.

5. Do percussion (hacking) around the lower leg for 15 seconds. Effleurage lightly.

6. Extend the leg over the pillow and move to the side. Effleurage from the ankle to the front of the pelvis 10 times.

7. Place your whole hand across the front and outside of the thigh, thumbs nearest your body. Knead by using close palm contact with fingers together to squeeze the leg in a push/pull action for 30 seconds. Effleurage deeply from knee to pelvis 5 times.

8. Do petrissage on the inner hamstrings of the back of the leg which can just be felt inside the knee; these and the groin muscles are gently pressed with the fingertips. Begin from the knee and proceed two-thirds of the way along the groin, at which point the muscles separate, and work back down for 30 seconds. Effleurage deeply 5 times.

9. Do percussion (hacking) all over the thigh for 15 seconds. Effleurage lightly then extend and stroke to the whole leg.

There is an obvious anatomical difference between male and female thighs, with those of men being more muscular and parallel, while women converge at the knee and have greater tension on the outside of thigh. You may have to go lightly on the front of well-muscled male thighs for comfort and especially light on a female partner's groin, which is sensitive around the time of menstruation.

Arm Massage

The nerves in the body are distributed in such a way that some of those which control the interior organs are directly related to those of the skin. This is particularly true of the chest organs and the skin on the arms. People who experience constriction around the heart often notice peculiar feelings in their arms first because the nervous energy to both areas originates from the same nerve 'root' in the spine. By what is known as 'reflex action' we can send the relaxing benefits of arm massage to the chest. In itself arm massage is very soothing, especially for those unable to accept full body massage.

1. Position yourself as for hand massage.
2. Effleurage by stroking from wrist to elbow 10 times, encircling the arm with both hands (Figure 27).
3. Petrissage softly, squeezing up and down the forearm for 30 seconds. (You are massaging the muscles which move the fingers and you may notice trembling in the hand.) Effleurage deeply 5 times.
4. To enable you to get to the upper arm comfortably for effleurage, try having your partner hold on to your shoulder, while you bend forward slightly (Figure 28). If this is not satisfactory, the arm can lie flat along the couch, or you can raise it with one hand while the other strokes it. Effleurage from elbow to shoulder 10 times.
5. Knead with both hands close on to the arm, squeezing the muscles away from the bone. Continue up into the shoulder muscle, for 30 seconds. Effleurage deeply 5 times.

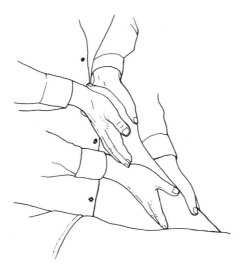

Fig. 27

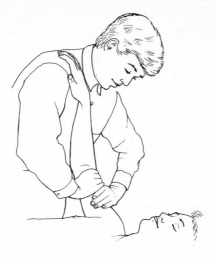

Fig. 28

6. Do percussion (hacking) all around the arm for 15 seconds. Effleurage lightly.

Be careful when treating the upper arm that you don't press on the 'funny bone', where the ulnar nerve, which supplies the little finger side of the forearm and hand, passes behind the inner side of the elbow joint. It is not at all amusing for your partner as they relax and, from your point of view, if they are holding on to your shoulder at that moment, you may receive an involuntary clip on the ear!

Chest Massage

Women have sensitive breast tissue covering the pectoral muscles, the important arm movers which lie over the chest wall. Men can also find direct pressure on the chest uncomfortable, so this massage is concerned with drainage points in the circulatory system rather than with the muscles. When these points are very active during menstruation or acute illnesses like influenza, partners may find chest massage unacceptable; cupping, percussion or frictions over the ribs may, however, relieve congested chests.

1. Have your partner lie facing upwards; put a small pillow under their shoulders.

2. Continue the arm effleurage stroke, with your inside hand, gliding along the chest just beneath the collarbone and on to the breastbone. Make the return stroke to the armpit slightly stronger. Repeat 4 times.
3. Walk your fingertips or knuckles from the breastbone to the armpit, in this direction only. With male partners you may use the heel of the hand as well as the fingers. Repeat 4 times. Effleurage as at 2.
4. Support the arm and move it gently around the shoulder, lightly stretching it away from the body to release tension in the chest muscles.
5. After massaging both sides of the chest, ask your partner to breathe deeply while you compress their rib cage on exhalation. Place your hands flat against the outsides of the chest and squeeze *gently*, releasing to allow a deeper breath in.

You can combine chest massage with massage of the back by having your partner lie on their side. It is then possible to treat half of the back with the shoulders and rib cage; try the cupping percussion to help with congestion inside the chest.

Massage of the Abdomen

We are cautions about being touched around the abdomen, perhaps because it contains our vital organs and seems a very intimate part of our body, or perhaps it just feels relatively unprotected. The abdomen is indeed a highly nervous area and, combined with these other considerations, it is not surprising that some partners find this massage unbearably ticklish. You might find that you are creating more tension that relaxation by working in this area, but persevere because it is a very beneficial massage.

Experiment by practising on your own abdomen to develop an acceptable touch for your partner.

1. Stand to the side of your partner close to the couch. Effleurage around the abdomen 10 times in a clockwise direction. Stroke gently but not too lightly, otherwise you will stimulate reflexes in the abdomen.
2. *Cross-over:* this is a combined effleurage/pressure stroke which relaxes the waist muscles. Fold your arms and place

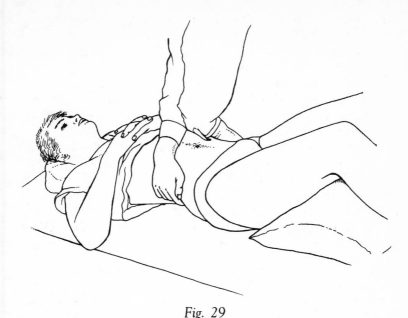

Fig. 29

your palms against and slightly underneath the waist (Figure 29); squeeze and lift up the waist, then let the body slip between the hand as you pass across the abdomen. Fold your arms alternately one above the other and repeat 6 times. Effleurage.

3. Knead the centre of the abdomen with fingers stretched from thumbs, up and down from the ribs to the front of the pelvis 6 times. (Go more lightly as you near the bladder which is in the lower abdomen.) Effleurage.

4. *Scoop*: this is another combined effleurage/pressure stroke which helps the posture of the abdomen. Use the edge and palm of your hands alternately to make firm waves from the lower to the upper abdomen 20 times (Figure 30). This stroke encourages the lower back muscles to relax and tips the pelvis backwards; the abdominal contents, which are, dragged down by gravity, are repositioned and abdominal congestion is relieved. Effleurage.

5. Repeat crossovers and effleurage as before 10 times.

Abdominal massage is recommended as an excellent self-massage. Women may find the scooping stroke 4 particularly

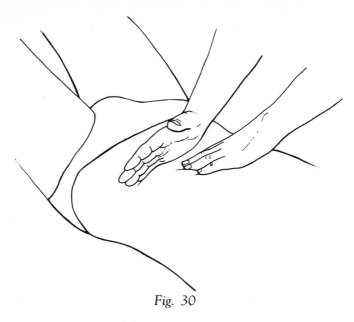

Fig. 30

helpful for menstrual pains when combined with low back massage. Massaging the abdomen can also help 'low spirits' when life feels like a burden, by stimulating the nerve endings in the abdominal plexus, and raising energy.

Neck Massage (lying down)

Our neck keeps our head high but it is also an important bridge between the brain and the rest of the body. Considering the extreme tensions from which the neck can suffer, it is remarkable that communications are so good. This is because the neck is a very flexible and resilient structure – as long as its muscles are sufficiently relaxed. Anxieties and worries increase the neck's tension and our shoulders tend to rise as problems mount.

1. Have your partner facing upwards and take up position at the head. Make all the movements in this massage very slowly, and explain to your partner clearly what you intend to do.
2. To do effleurage, first roll the head gently to the left side,

like a ball, not raising it. Use your right hand to stroke evenly up and down the neck on to the shoulder, 10 times. Roll the head to the other side and repeat.

3. Returning the head to the left side, place your fingers under the neck and your thumb along its side. Knead squeeze gently by pushing and releasing the hand against the neck (Figure 31). Avoid pressing directly with the thumb. Do this for 30 seconds and then repeat to the other side of the neck.

4. Place the head in the centre. Using both hands, repeat the squeezing stroke from the base of the skull up and down the back of the neck.

5. *Stretching*:
   a. roll the head to the right with your left hand, then, crossing your forearms, place your right hand against the left shoulder (Figure 32). Ask your partner to take a long inhalation. As they exhale, slowly and evenly stretch the head towards the right shoulder, for the duration of the out-breath. If their chin goes well towards the shoulder, the stretch is quite sufficient. Very slowly roll the head to the other side and repeat.
   b. support the head in both hands and stretch forwards.

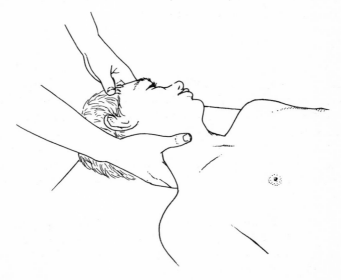

Fig. 31

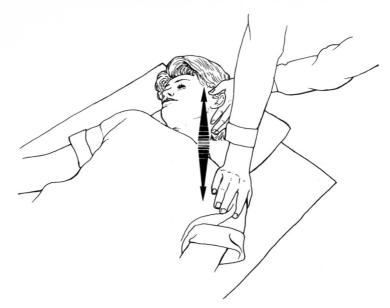

Fig. 32

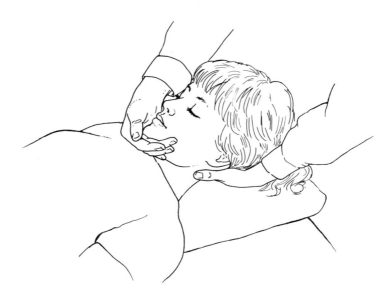

Fig. 33

The chin may almost touch the chest. Use the same breathing rhythm as for the previous stretch.

c. is a traction. Hold the whole head firmly but comfortably. As your partner exhales, draw the head away from the body (Figure 33). This may seem very adventurous but is in fact a simple movement! The stretch relies on the stronger downward force exerted by the exhalation rather than on your 'pull', so there is less actual force used than in the previous stretches.

6. Effleurage lightly around the head, neck and shoulders. You may like to improvise a face massage as your partner relaxes from the stretches.

The stretches are safe. You will feel a 'give' while stretching your partner's neck muscles which is due to the loosening effect of prior kneading. Providing you keep the movements slow, your partner will always be in control of the stretch; however, out of respect for bodies over fifty years of age, where suppleness may be declining, don't stretch middle-aged partners without supervision.

When someone has an established arthritic condition which has affected the wrists or hands, it may also have damaged the stability of the joints of the neck; in this case your can offer the following, very gentle, version of neck massage with your partner sitting upright.

Neck Massage (seated)

Neck massage can also be given with partners in the sitting position. This has the advantage that pressure from tensions are easily drawn downwards and the posture of the neck and head improved. This can be a very spontaneous massage, done almost anywhere, and has converted many sceptics to the pleasure of whole body treatments.

1. Standing behind, do effleurage from the sides of the head down the neck and over the shoulders to the upper arms. Repeat 6 times.
2. Do light petrissage on the ridge of the shoulders. Use the thumbs, resting the fingers over the shoulders, moving from the centre to the outside edges for 30 seconds. Effleurage as before.

3. Hold your partner's forehead in the palm of your right hand and pinch up and down the back of the neck with your left hand for 30 seconds. Repeat, changing your hands around. Effleurage as before.
4. Allow the head to rest back against your abdomen. Effleurage from the forehead to the temples, and from the chin to the temples, 6 times.
5. Petrissage, using the fingertips to circle lightly over the face (very gently near the eyes) for 30 seconds. Effleurage as before.
6. Use percussion (tapotement), with your fingertips drumming all over the face for 15 seconds. Effleurage.
7. Replace the head in the upright position and, still supporting it with one hand, effleurage one side 6 times from the head through the neck and shoulders to the upper arm. Repeat on the other side.
8. Ask your partner to fully support their neck, and repeat effleurage with both hands, 6 times each stroke becoming lighter and lighter.

Conclusion

Having completed a sequence of massage, cover your partner over and keep them warm so as to continue their sense of being cared for. A massaged partner might be drowsy or asleep or may want to talk; you should be available for their time of transition back to 'normality' but it may be that you feel the need to withdraw. Professionals recognize this possibility by giving a fifty-minute massage in an hour's treatment so as to allow a few minutes for a satisfactory ending. In a busy practice it is easy to forget how valuable this time can be for both so it is a habit you can adopt from the outset.

SPECIAL MASSAGES – MOBILIZING

After completing the strokes of a treatment, you can magnify your partner's sense of relaxation by 'mobilizing'. This involves moving each joint slowly through its natural range of movement, with co-operation but not assistance from your partner. Simply allowing someone else to move our body is not easy and, even when apparently willing, partners are often unable to 'let go' completely. This is an indication of how tensions sometimes represent an investment of energy which can get 'locked up' in the body. By patiently waiting and moving sensitively, rather than forcing, you will eventually be able to move their body with lessening resistance.

For the limbs

The arm and leg joints are designed to move freely, and they have lubricating fluids to ensure smoothness. Movement normally occurs from muscles pulling across the joint, and when we mobilize our partner our hands take the place of their muscles. For maximum benefit move the joints the way they seem to want to go and just a little further.

Example: Support the elbow in your palm and hold their hand in the other. Slowly bend the elbow, pausing when you feel your partner 'helping', until it is fully flexed and then extend it straight. Repeat until the elbow joint opens and closes with ease. Notice that the elbow flexes with the palm turned up or down, and mobilize in both directions.

For the shoulder

Anxiety and monotonous posture severely reduce what should be 360° mobility of the shoulder: can your partner swing their right arm over the head, take the left arm behind their back and, bending the elbow, touch their fingers? If not, the following movement will be beneficial:

1. Ask your partner to lie sideways, with a pillow under their head and their top leg bending forwards for steadiness.
2. Lightly massage the arm and side of the neck.
3. Thread your arm through theirs to support its weight. Clasp the shoulder between both hands (Figure 34).
4. Move the shoulder up and down, then forwards and backwards. As your partner relaxes and their arm feels heavier, begin a circular movement. If you can get your fingertips under the shoulder-blade, this will release more tension.

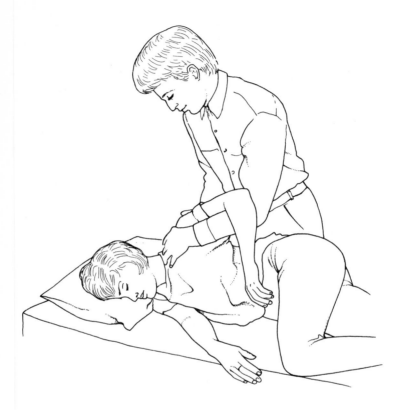

Fig. 34

5. Replace the arm, and effleurage before asking your partner to turn over slowly. Repeat movements to the other side.

Many people find this a soporific treatment; if your partner falls asleep by the end of the massage to the second shoulder, they probably need to; cover them over and stay close by.

For the hip

Stiffness in the hip is accompanied by increased buttock tension on the affected side, which can be observed with your partner facing downwards. This treatment also helps with pains in the leg which have origins in the lower back;

52

for example, the unpleasant sensation radiating down the back of the leg, known as sciatica, when the pressure affects the great sciatic nerve.

1. Ask your partner to lie face down. Place a small pillow under the abdomen and a large pillow under the feet. check the tension in the buttocks.
2. Put one hand flat against the upper thigh while slowly raising and lowering the foot (Figure 35). When there is a problem in the hip, the knee joint will not move easily.
3. Push hard on to the thigh with your palm as you flex the knee to 90°. Increase the pressure on the thigh, then lower the foot slowly, releasing the pressure as the foot touches the pillow.
4. Repeat 3 times. Check for reduced tension in the buttock, and treat both legs until equally relaxed. (For one-sided tension, place a pillow under the pelvic bone on the opposite side.)

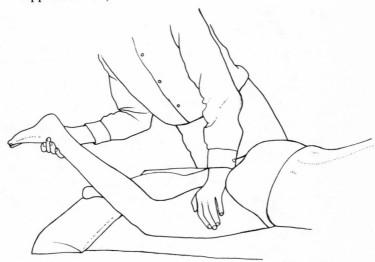

Fig. 35

For the neck

The joints of the neck have a wide range of movement, unlike the rest of the spine which has to accommodate and support the chest and pelvis. The graceful curves of the neck are easily forfeited to fixed occupational postures, however, and this mobilization is an attempt to remind us of the neck's full potential.

1. Ask your partner to lie towards the top of the couch so that their head and neck extends beyond the end of the couch, and support the head with your hands. This is very testing of the trust between you; if the head should slip from your hands, your partner would probably recover control but their neck muscles might never forgive you.

   (For the reassurance of both parties, you may place a smaller table under the head so the distance below is less but still enough to allow movement. Before you begin the mobilization, read through the whole text, then give your complete attention to the movements.)
2. *Very slowly* move the head up and down and from side to side (Figure 36). If you are successful, you will feel the head increasingly heavy as the neck relaxes.
3. Lower the head a little and hold it quite still (Figure 37); rotate it to each side and while it is fully turned, lower it a little further. This is the most helpful movement so don't rush it.
4. Repeat all the movements, checking that your partner still feels comfortable, then support the head to allow recovery back down on to the couch. Place the head on a small pillow and ask your partner to breathe deeply.

Mobilizations can be very helpful after injury or illness to bring confidence back to movements. After a period of immobility, even everyday movements can be painful, whereas your mobilizations should be painless. Your partner may feel disoriented after giving you responsibility for their movements, so be aware of possible unsteadiness as they get up, and caution them to move slowly at first.

Gain experience of applying the mobilizations on your fittest partners, who can join you in a spirit of investigation! If you consider a deeper movement might be of special help to someone, double check with them first for contra-indications. It is unlikely that you could cause harm but you may find all your earlier relaxing work undone if a partner is unprepared for deeper massage.

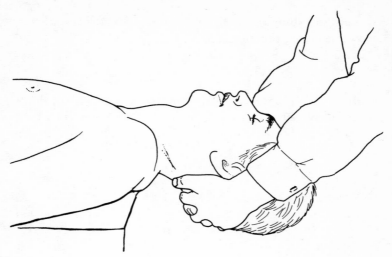

Fig. 36

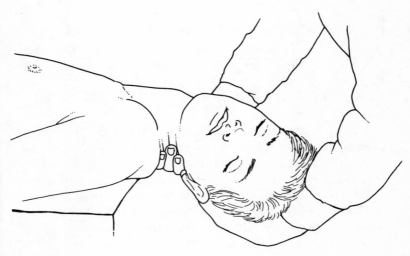

Fig. 37

REVIEW

Before going on to look at the specific applications of massage, let's review your practice so far:

Are you enjoying the massage as much as your partners appear to be?
So that your energy keeps pace with your enthusiasm, don't spend much more than an hour treating someone. Too long a session can become debilitating for you both and, if you increase the number of your treatments, you won't be able to give everyone a very long session.

Are you learning about the body with each massage?
During even the briefest treatment your partner is offering you a lesson and an opportunity to understand how the body works. Without making your partner feel like a 'specimen', adapt your treatment plan according to any changes in their condition.

Are you aware of any emotional strain connected with giving massages?
Even if you intend to steer clear of your partner's life-problems, there may be occasions when your own mood makes you vulnerable to another's distress. How will you handle this? If your treatments seem to be going well you may not have connected fluctuations in your own emotions with the act of giving massage.

Tiredness can be as much a sign of this kind of strain as over-exertion, and you should realize that your emotional muscles need as much conditioning as those which you use to perform massage.

Professionals learn to dissociate themselves from one person's problems to the next, through an appointment system which encourages exclusive concentration on the specific problem at hand. In a more casual atmosphere, it may still help you to follow other formal procedures such as thorough hand-washing, or making a few notes on your reactions to a session. In the longer term, it is advisable not to 'carry' your partner's emotional material even when it may feel manageable; partners who seem to need more out of massage than you are able to give should be referred on to experienced practitioners.

Is your practice growing?
The more massage you give, the clearer it will become which part of the body or aspect of the strokes you are naturally drawn towards. Partners often feel in need of particular attention, (eg 'My shoulders give me trouble') which is acknowledged even though we recognize the necessity of treating the whole body. Without speaking diagnostically, make it known to partners that you are developing an interest in treating common sites of tension. In certain situations, this may be the only route to access deeper but treatable problems which general massages fail to relieve.

6

What Massage Does

NOW THAT YOU have some experience of the methods, both you and your partner will have begun to realize why massage has such a deserved reputation as a *therapy*. The permission we give others to massage us is not given lightly, however, and passively submitting to being touched is not the same as allowing ourselves to be *moved*; it is the establishment of trust and co-operation which allows the strokes of massage to relieve both physical and emotional discomfort.

Measurable benefits have been well researched by practitioners: because of the persuasiveness of the muscles throughout the body, their skilful manipulation assists the circulation in the blood and lymphatic vessels, stimulates the organs of digestion and elimination, and improves the performance of the lungs and skin.

As the muscles themselves improve in tone, so do the nerves which supply them, to the spinal cord and back to the brain. The nerves provide the stimulus for motion and sensibility and are extremely alert to the atmosphere inside and outside the body. It is not easy to evaluate massage psychologically except in that most people agree it is a potentially pleasurable experience.

Let us now look at a real example of how massage played a deeper role in helping with an emotional problem.

A CASE STUDY

An older adult who reported a sudden onset of 'dizziness' was seen by her physician who diagnosed high blood pressure. Although the patient had been the same weight over many years the treatment prescribed was to lose weight quickly by dieting.

After no change in weight or blood pressure, a sympathetic friend made arrangements for massage treatments. The initial session revealed severe tension in her neck and shoulders. During the session, the patient hinted at an emotional crisis involving the reappearance of another person in her life and the strain it was causing. It was a painful but just bearable situation to which the restrictive diet for her 'weight problem' was felt as a further affliction. With reassurance that raised blood pressure was not unnatural where there was emotional strain, the shoulders became much more massageable.

As massage treatments continued and a near normal diet resumed, the situation showed some signs of being resolved and her blood pressure dropped. The sessions were punctuated by considerable distress, however, when the patient spoke of the background to the crisis. Eventually she was able to speak the unsaid to her friend and life gradually became more peaceful.

Perhaps this could be considered a straightforward case except that the patient was as much concerned with her reaction to the crisis as to its cause. What was massage able to offer this person?

1. Sometimes a medical diagnosis can be a welcome dis-
   traction from a problem, but here it only emphasized an
   aspect of the problem and in a punitive way. The massage
   highlighted the tension in the neck and shoulders as being
   connected with emotional pressure, and thus the alarm of
   the original diagnosis (which itself was contributing to the
   emotional strain) was minimized.
2. The treatment of the shoulders and arms allowed freer
   circulation between the extremities and the chest (which
   tends to become restricted with unhappiness or anger).
   Nervous controls shared by the chest and arms were also
   influenced, so that deeper breathing, a reliever of pressure,
   was induced.
3. The treatments enabled the person to use the supportive
   atmosphere of the massage treatment to express herself.
   This is quite different from a response in conversation

or analysis in that it was accepted that the problem had become physically manifested in the body. Her dialogue with the practitioner was able to move between the verbal and the muscular according to her feelings; where words failed, focus returned to the muscles, and when tension was greatest, words came.

FEAR

The case study above illustrates how fear, often from past experience, influences emotional life. When we are initially frightened, our body sets up special safeguards which are entirely defensive. Unless we have become stiff with fright, we are usually being prepared for almost *heroic* action; when circumstances frustrate activity, acute tension is produced.

In many 'civilized' circumstances, action may be unacceptable or may even provoke greater strain (especially interpersonal), so that we often chose a milder, displacing response, such as *eating*.

In one sense this is curious, since we have little power of digestion when afraid; undigested foods are not absorbed but give rise to substances which are circulated around the body and can ultimately lead to the tensing of muscles and stiffening of joints characteristic of rigid fear.

In the short term a sense of stiffness and unease brings a genuine feeling of distress, as we enter a vicious cycle where the original problem is easily obscured. From a dietary point of view the option to eat may be a variation on primitive chewing, to which 'chewing gum' and smoking may be heirs. (If food is taken in such conditions, it would appear from the study of digestion that *slow* eating is less harmful.)

If what we are seeking from eating is reassurance, the safe touch of massage may provide the answer. The contact needs to be genuine rather than expert, though it can take time to get used to having someone else 'handle' our stress. The massager is then in a position to shift our awareness from frustration or bewilderment to a more grounded experience of how our body is coping with the situation.

TENSIONS AND POSTURE

The tensions created by fear also distort our posture. Sometimes we respond to unsolvable problems by pushing our chin
forward, pulling our arms tight against our sides, or twisting
our pelvis in an attempt to draw away. In similar situations
animals pretend to grow in size, but humans usually end up
diminished. Unreleased tension causes shortening of the spine,
which begins to show in an expanded abdomen, flattening of
the feet, and a backward tilt of the head. As well as relieving
this tension, massage is able to remould our posture.

Improved posture releases us from a subtle cycle of strain.
If a taller person stoops, does this make them appear more or
less threatening to people smaller than themselves? When we
draw back our pelvis when others come near, do we realize this
gives the impression that we are about to fall towards them?
Because we are using more effort to maintain such a posture,
we may convince our friends that we are relaxed, but sooner
or later it begins to hurt. Massagers are immediately aware of
inconsistent posture, and their treatments aim to challenge
the tension without removing it prematurely. It is as if we say
to ourselves: 'I feel anxious so I'll arch my back' but forget
that after a short time an arching back also creates anxiety.
It would be better to discover this with the help of massage
than to develop a chronic problem which has to be 'corrected'
by more drastic means.

The movements of massage create a sense of space within
our posture and give us the chance to reassess our reactions
to problems in life. They offer a way to poise amidst the many
stresses which surround us, allowing a more constructive use
of our muscles.

In an earlier chapter I described how massage is carried
out by the body on itself. Having begun to learn what your
additional massages can achieve, you are also increasing in
knowledge about the body. Your development in massage will
be enhanced by combining the confidence which comes from
knowledge with your natural ability to treat. Everything you
discover about how massage benefits an injury or illness will
be an inspiration in your work to raise healthy bodies to an
even healthier level.

7

Techniques

TECHNIQUES ARE TREATMENTS whose applications have consistently improved a condition or relieved a problem where general treatments have failed. Techniques are often mysterious, glamorous or personalized, and are available on very expensive courses. Some techniques highlight the causes of problems and can explain living anatomy better than texts, while others demonstrate the gifted skills of their innovators.

Techniques have reputations which seem to hold out a promise of success to practitioner and patient. Within the professions there can be controversy over which school has the correct 'angle' on a particular technique and this move towards specialization, while intending to benefit the patient, can reduce the human element in treatments.

Successful techniques are the *discoveries* of dedicated practitioners but often we cannot be sure whether a technique represents the culmination of a person's work or merely an effective stage in a new direction. This has been disconcerting for certain schools of therapy, since many famous and inspired founders have been unable to explain satisfactorily their special methods. Often their students do a much better job, yet we might wonder if an innovator would still be emphasizing a particular method a hundred years after he first demonstrated it, or whether he would have moved on.

As you continue in massage you will probably discover your own techniques. I would like you to use this chapter for experimentation, rather than create the impression that you have so much more to learn. The techniques described illustrate a particular quality of the body, and the skill of its practitioners. Experiment with them and perhaps incorporate some of the ideas into your own methods. Even if you are not inspired, still try some of these techniques just to get an idea of what a partner might experience at the hands of a specialist. You will not be able to claim the expertise of their well-trained exponents but by continuous application you may arrive at the principle in the mind of the technique's originator.

I confidently predict that you will produce your own successful innovations as your practice grows: keep notes of your intuitive techniques and watch them develop.

AROMATHERAPY

Aromatherapy involves massage using oil which has been blended with the essence of a plant. The essences themselves are a little oily, very fragrant, and usually too concentrated to be used neat. They are extracted by a variety of methods according to whether the fruit, leaf or stem of the plant is used. Vast amounts of raw materials are required to produce even a small amount of essential oil, and their harvesting and lengthy production make them expensive.

Essential oils have been used therapeutically since biblical times. The discovery of their chemical composition in recent years has brought about an increasing use of synthetic scents, but these have become the perfumes of the cosmetics industry. Though incomparable, the new essences were far cheaper to produce and their high alcohol content meant they could be kept indefinitely. The current trend back towards more natural products has fortunately led to a revival in demand for true essential oils, and their original role is being rediscovered.

Research has shown that essential oils possess the medicinal properties associated with herbs, are antiseptic and capable of adjusting a person's mood via the olfactory nerves. Although the oils are highly concentrated, they are without side effects if used properly, although a person's reaction to treatment may be more emotional than anticipated. The massages are given in part rather than a whole body treatment, with periods of calm effleurage to allow a partner to appreciate the fragrance of the oil.

For the Face

Oil – *Lemongrass*
(I recommend you buy a ready-blended oil; you may add a few drops of essence to base vegetable oil for experimentation but this is not the same as blending.)

1. Stand or sit at your partner's head within easy reach of the face. A towel or head band can be used to clear away the hair.
2. Place a few drops of blended oil on your hand and spread it lightly on to the face. Effleurage the face from the chin to the temples and across the forehead 10 times.
3. Make circular strokes with your fingertips on the cheeks for 10 seconds. Effleurage towards the ears.
4. Do similar strokes along the jaw line to its hinges beside the ears. Reverse and, reaching the chin, continue around the mouth, moving the lips but without opening the mouth. Repeat 6 times. Effleurage.
5. Stroke the rims of the eye sockets, one-finger effleurage, firmer on the upper rim, 3 times.
6. Look for tension lines on the forehead – horizontal, vertical or both – and rub at right angles for 10 seconds. Effleurage deeply upwards and outwards.
7. Hold the ear lobes and pull gently down and away from the head 3 times.
8. Percuss the whole face with tapotement – fingertips drumming – avoiding the eyes.
9. Effleurage the face from the chin to the temples and across the forehead 10 times, getting very light to finish.
10. 'Comb' through the hair, lightly scratching the scalp. Take good handfuls of hair and squeeze or pull until the scalp stretches 3 times.

You will not be able to return to stroke the face after hair pulling, so complete the treatment by effleuraging the shoulders.

Although we strive to maintain the hygiene of our face, from a massager's point of view it really is a neglected area of the body. Our fixed expressions keep the muscles of the face in tension over long periods, and the combination of polluted city-life and the effects of air-conditioning are very damaging to the skin. Neck tension further adds to the pressures which build up, especially around our eyes, impeding their circulation and drainage.

Women may confuse the deeper benefits of face massage with the 'facial' of beauty treatments, and many men will have missed the experience of the massage which used to go with the barber's shave. Revive face massage!

For the Back
(Stiffness and pain after activities, exertion etc.)

Oil – *Sage*
1. Before applying the oil, friction the whole back with palms and fingertips to create a good circulation (*hyperaemia*).
2. Stand at the head of your partner. Pour a teaspoonful of oil into your hands and apply to the whole back. (You may need more later according to the skin type.)
3. Do reverse effleurage 10 times, stroking down the centre of the back, and returning via the waist and sides of the chest to the armpit.
4. Using your fingertips, 'rake' all over the back.
5. Use the edge of your hands or knuckles to glide over the back at different angles.
6. Snatch at the skin, especially up around the shoulders. Effleurage deeply.
7. Twist the skin into an 'S' shape using your thumbs (Figure 38).
8. Pick up the skin and roll it between your thumbs and fingers from the upper to lower back and to the sides of the chest.
9. Repeat reverse effleurage, giving a deep stretch to the lower back, and on return draw the shoulders wide.
10. Cover your partner and keep them warm. Allow extra time for your partner to recover from an aromatherapy treatment.

Don't try to knead the muscles of the back using oil because you won't have enough control. Direct your strokes to the skin, toning it and increasing the circulation to the muscles underneath. When your partner is feeling tender from emotion or too much exertion, this 'skin-deep' technique is more

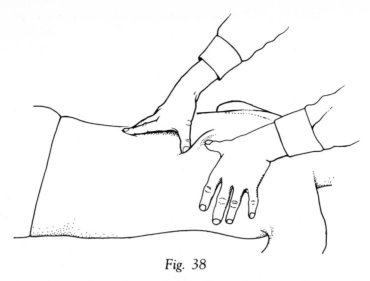

Fig. 38

acceptable and painless, while still conditioning the muscles underneath.

HYDROTHERAPY

Hydrotherapy is used in conjunction with massage. The effect of water on the body can dramatically relieve pain and redistribute the circulation and act as a tonic. Animals practise a form of hydrotherapy by licking their wounds and by immersing themselves in streams when injured. Father Kneipp, a nineteenth-century priest and healer, pioneered the use of hydrotherapy in his Bavarian clinic, and became famous for the success of his technique on many human disorders.

The benefits of water therapy come from the reaction of our warm-blooded bodies; brief applications of water of different temperatures on the skin usually have an opposite effect; cold water acts tonically on the body and is usually preferred to hot, but *how* cold depends on the individual's make-up. Slender people require cold only slightly beneath blood temperature, whereas substantial bodies react better to an extreme. Our alarm at the prospect of coming into contact with chilly water is based on the expectation of a *long immersion*. However, our bodies tolerate cold much more readily than too much heat, as babies and those who recover from freezing conditions remind us; overheating is much more dangerous for our systems. Hot treatments, which should be applied gradually, are used to soothe and relax and are especially effective on the back of the body.

The following examples of hydrotherapy are simply applied yet very effective for two common problems.

For muscle spasm and relief of pain
(e.g. the calf muscles)

It is difficult to relax the great tension of a muscle spasm due to the chemical and nervous conditions within the muscle at that time, which make it hypersensitive. Even if we can get a moderate pressure on to the affected part, it may still be insufficient. We could try more pressure and attempt to replace the first pain by a greater pain – like biting on a toothache – but we may injure ourselves more. The following method is a much safer way of bringing relief:

1. Have one bowl of very hot water and one of cold. Keep a hot kettle and a bag of ice nearby to 'top-up'. Soak a face flannel in each; apply the wrung out hot cloth for 30 seconds, then the cold for 30 seconds. Repeat six times, re-soaking the cloth between applications.

   (After the initial hot and cold, the temperature will *feel* less extreme and you can add from the kettle and ice bag after 3 times.)
2. Massage the muscle for 3 minutes, using deep effleurage. Cover and keep warm.

This hydrotherapy works well on the limbs and neck; trunk muscles, especially on the back, respond better to short, hot immersions in a bath: 3–5 minutes before and after the massage.

For varicosity of the lower leg

The venous blood, returning to the heart near the surface of the body in soft-walled vessels, can suffer impediments. The blood in the legs has the added resistance of gravity to overcome, and when pressures are great in the abdomen, or during pregnancy, the veins stretch and the blood 'queues' rather than flows – the veins swell and the legs ache.

This technique provides a helpful effleurage, which does not pressurize a painful vein.

1. Sit in a warm bath with your legs out of the water. Use a cold hand shower (or have a friend pour cold water) from the ankle to the knee but not back down, at least 12 times (Figure 39).
2. Dry the body but only wrap the legs in the towel. Rest with pillows under the lower legs, knees bent for 10 minutes.
3. Give back and abdominal massage to relieve the strain on varicose veins.

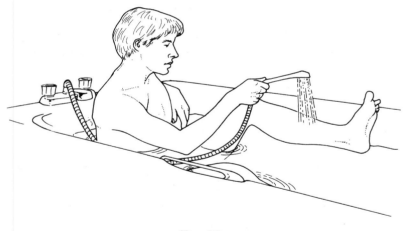

Fig. 39

OSTEOPATHY

Osteopathy is a form of manipulative treatment, conceived in the nineteenth century by Andrew Taylor-Still in Kansas, USA. Taylor-Still was a compassionate observer of the structure of bodies and he contended that our skeletal posture strongly influences the functioning of the other systems, particularly the nerves. Osteopathic techniques concentrate on releasing 'lesions', areas of abnormal tension, especially around the spinal column.

Osteopaths have a rigorous training to become specialists in muscle, joint and bone disorders. The technique has the reputation for equally vigorous application, but in recent years the popular image of 'back-cracking' has given way to a more gentle style.

The technique described is of the milder approach and relies on the co-operation of your partner. It can be used on any of the limb joints: after an injury has healed leaving stiffness; when a job or recreation results in one side of the body becoming lighter than the other; or as a deeper relaxing movement after a whole body massage.

For the hip joint

1. Have your partner lie flat on their back. Fold one knee as close as possible up to the chest. Repeat with the other leg

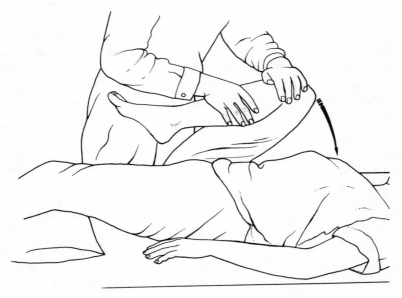

Fig. 40

and compare the flexion at the hip. (Ask if your partner confirms your observation.)

2. After relaxing both legs down, fold the 'stiffer' leg up and gently press it as far as you can towards the chest. Pause.
3. Ask your partner to push steadily against your pressure, while you resist equally so that you counteract their effort (Figure 40). Hold for 5 seconds.
4. Ask your partner to relax slowly. As their pressure decreases, slowly follow through, pressing their leg closer to the chest. Lean against the leg rather than pushing with your hands, and expect the joint to release a little.
5. Re-starting from this improved position, repeat the technique twice more. It should be painless and your partner will be surprised at how much they can 'give'. You are not forcing the hip but rather guiding the leg into space created by releasing the hip's antagonistic muscles.

If your partner has a rheumatic condition of their joint, you may not achieve much improvement in position and they will feel pain on pressure. If you have their confidence, however, you can do the technique without 'following through', which will help relax the joint and perhaps relieve the pain of stiffness. If, however, they have had a hip joint replacement, beware! Forced flexions of an artificial joint can result in dislocation. Simply supporting the leg, with knee flexed, while your partner moves ('active movement') will help loosen up the muscles with safety.

POLARITY THERAPY

Polarity Therapy is a subtle technique, which regards the body as an energy system, with 'positive' and 'negative' aspects:

- + at the head;
- − at the feet;
- + to the front;
- − to the back.

The therapist places a polarizing hand (+ = right) over a

partner's uncomfortable area and, using little or no contact, produces a balancing effect.

Randolph Stone (1890–1983), an Austrian who lived in the USA and India, is accredited as the 'father' of Polarity Therapy, which he described as a blending of oriental techniques.

Polarity is especially useful when someone's muscles are so tense as to make massage difficult, or when they are impossible to touch, for instance, if they are in a plaster cast. The use of the technique in chronic tension can have a strong emotional effect on partners. I used the technique on someone who had been 'trying' various treatments over some years. After ten minutes of Polarity (his eyes were closed and he was unable to see where my hands were positioned), he spoke of unlocking sensations in his head. 'I don't know what you were doing, but I couldn't take much more of that !'

It's a good idea to have some Polarity treatment yourself so that you become aware of the releasing sensations which can occur if you intend to use it on a partner.

Head cradle

This is a preparatory treatment to more complex Polarities.

1. Have your partner lie flat on their back. Place your palms along the sides of their head, the left hand slightly higher.
2. Point your index fingers towards the chest. Your hands should take the shape of the head, softly enclosing but not really holding (Figure 41).
3. Be relaxed in yourself without trying to feel particularly calm; keep your mind open and associate freely. Don't ask your partner to relax, but occasionally suggest they take a deep breath.
4. Offer your presence to your partner, simply being with them, accepting rather than trying to change their condition.
5. Initially, limit a session to five minutes until you get used to this technique. Take time for your own deep breathing afterwards.

Polarity Therapy is particularly concerned with the physical

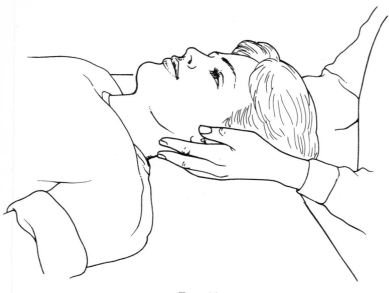

Fig. 41

discomforts which arise with psychological problems. Do not be surprised at your partner's responses which can accompany release of tension: sighing, coughing, laughing or crying. Be sure you feel able to accept spontaneous emotional expression before you decide to use Polarity on your partner.

REFLEXOLOGY

Early Egyptian and Chinese civilizations practised Reflexology, sometimes called 'Zone Therapy'. The basis of this technique is that reflex points mapped out on the feet and hands are related to different areas of the body. As we know from everyday experience, the soles of the feet and palms are richly supplied with nerve endings but these are not the same as the reflexes.

The technique is thought to be derived from Chinese acupuncture theory, which is very humanistic compared to rational Western medicine and conceives of a body-energy which includes the personality. The reflexes extend from the extremities to the top of the head along 'meridians' or pathways containing physical and emotional elements of health. By applying pressure on the reflex points, the reflexologist releases congestion along the meridians and improves the functioning of the body organs.

The spinal reflexes

If your partner's spinal muscles are in spasm or you are unsure about treating a 'bad' back, try this technique:

1. Have your partner stand sideways, then lie down and compare the silhouette of their foot with that of the spine. I have always found this to correspond (Figure 42).

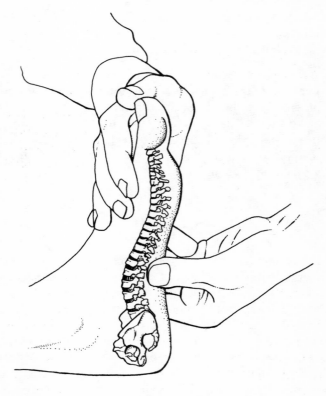

Fig. 42

For example, a long arch of the foot will be reflected in the lumbar spine; a strong curve over the base of the big toe is usually seen as a pronounced curve of the thoracic spine.

2. Place a pillow under the knees and the ankles so that the feet extend. Steady the foot by lightly holding the toes, and effleurage the instep with the thumb or heel of your hand, with even pressure in both directions.
3. Using the edge of your thumb, trace along the instep and feel for hard points, 'knots' or 'crunches'. These points are usually unexpectedly painful for back sufferers and will reflect as the tightest areas of the spinal column.
4. Using a flatter part of your thumb, keep a steady circling pressure on a painful point as if to rub it away. You will gradually be able to increase pressure, and the pain will lessen. There are normally at least two such strongly sensitive points along the spinal reflex. Spend up to two minutes on each point.
5. Effleurage the instep and treat the other foot.

You may wash your partner's feet in warm water before the treatment, and your hands in cold water afterwards. If during the massage your hands begin to feel uncomfortable, stop and shake them; this will be a refreshing pause and helpful to your partner. Many people fall asleep during Reflexology, so be careful to awaken them by softly calling their name, or gently touching their hand.

SHIATSU

Shiatsu is a Japanese word for finger-pressure massage. Practitioners use their thumbs, elbows and heels to disperse tensions throughout the body. Many Japanese use the services of the visiting Shiatsu therapist, and it is common for members of the family to practise on each other.

Shiatsu is known to effect calming influences on hypertensions, while people too low in tension can be energized. Many people find the technique useful for pain relief, and it demonstrates something we already know by instinct – pressure on one tender spot often releases a wider area of tension. The meridians of the Chinese system are thought to operate in Shiatsu.

For the shoulder

Stand behind your seated partner and ask for some movement in a stiff shoulder. Squeeze gently around the shoulder joint and scapula. It may be that your partner is tender or numb around the shoulder. In regular massage, you would try to loosen up the area with petrissage; instead try the following:

1. Using thumb pressure, move around the whole shoulder, probing deeply. It is very likely that you will discover one or more unexpectedly painful points.
2. Place your thumb (or both thumbs together on a strong shoulder) directly on a point (Figure 43). Ask your partner to breathe out slowly as you press directly into the point for approximately 10 seconds. Release the pressure gradually as your partner inhales.

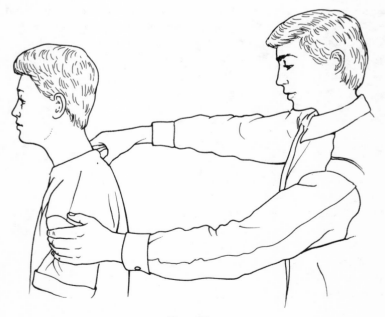

Fig. 43

3. You should explain the foregoing to prepare your partner for such a direct pressure. The formerly painful point will desensitize as they breathe out, and you can encourage them by breathing out in unison. It may also help if they visualize the pain being pressed out of their body.
4. Repeat twice more on other points around the same area.
5. Mobilize the shoulder gently and ask if your partner observes the freer movement.

For fatigue

This Shiatsu combines with the principles of Reflexology for its benefits:

1. Have your partner lie face downwards on a padded floor, a small pillow under their feet which should be 12 inches apart.
2. Stand, facing away and delicately place your heels on to the soles of their feet (Figure 44).
3. Adding pressure gradually, knead the feet, transferring your weight from foot to foot, for a maximum of 10 minutes.
4. Wrap the feet up to keep them warm, and invite your partner to move into a comfortable position for further relaxation.

It may be a good idea on the first treatment to wash the feet

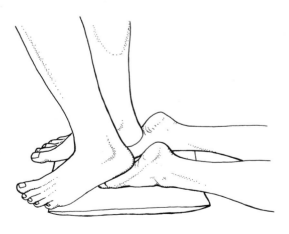

Fig. 44

in warm water first to assist the circulation. This will supple the soles and might offset the tendency for cramp in the instep due to your pressure being unrelieved. If cramp does occur, stop immediately, extend the big toe, and ask your partner to breathe deeply before trying to continue.

You may have heard of a massage technique which involves walking up the *entire body* from the feet, to include the spine; this is a wonderful experience but not recommended without *expert supervision*. I was introduced to it by a six stone Indonesian, so skilful she could walk from one body to the next!

8

Special Massages for Injuries

INJURIES ARE PART of everyday life – they record our over-exertions. Sometimes we don't notice an injury, like an old bruise which can't be explained, whereas a bone fracture, though rarely fatal, can become one of life's major inconveniences. Injuries are traumatic, in that our consciousness registers a reaction to any assault; when we experience this we are said to be 'in shock'.

Unlike our illnesses, which often recur, we make spectacularly complete recovery from most injuries. Even people trained to regard childbirth as a disease, marvel at the body's powers of self-repair from injury. While sophisticated accident and emergency units in hospitals provide expert care and accurate monitoring, their ultra-sterile and impersonal atmosphere does not accelerate the healing process.

Even the most devastating injuries are self-repairing, given minimum caring circumstances. Our nervous systems are so sensitive that by the time we are aware of a cut to the skin, for example, our body has already begun its repairing process. Few medicines have any positive influence on injuries, and the fractured bone – though sometimes requiring the skill of surgery for alignment – heals and makes itself stronger without any further attention.

Injuries happen to most of us, but apparently to some more than others. We cannot insure our health against injury yet they do seem to occur with a certain predictability: unfit bodies cope less with strain; tiredness and tension make us vulnerable to even minor exertion; an unbalanced diet can lead to weakness; carelessness often invites self-damage.

Our discussion will begin by describing the theoretical aspects of injury to the soft tissues of the body and go on to suggest ways in which massage can improve the conditions for healing.

If you are inspired towards the treatment and management of injuries, study of an up-to-date 'Pocket First Aid' by the Red Cross Society, or equivalent, is essential.

WHAT IS AN INJURY?

Our reaction to being injured often relates to how much inconvenience it creates. For treatment purposes, injuries can be categorized into two groups: 'Trivial', where damage is slight and recovery comes from simple resting; and 'Serious', in which there is destruction or discontinuity of tissue, producing disability.

Trivial

This category often refers to situations as much as to damage, where we assume that our injury is insignificant because of its simple cause. Also, our minor reactions are not always easy to assess; usually there is mild stiffness and some inflammation but if this diminishes after twenty-four hours, we feel a recovery has been made.

Many trivial injuries are caused by over use of the body, and even if the pressure to use does not relent, interruption and rest usually keep problems at bay. Recurring, *seemingly* trivial injuries, like the 'bad back', require investigation both of the condition and of the circumstances which provoke it.

Serious

Initially trivial injury can develop into serious injury. Otherwise it will be apparent from the outset that swelling or loss of blood and greater pain indicates that some severe damage has occurred. 'Serious' does not denote more life-threatening; in fact, vigorous reaction to injury demonstrates that the body is in full healthy response. More *time* will be required for healing, and this will give the opportunity to apply the appropriate treatments to optimize the body's effort.

WHAT HAPPENS DURING INJURY?

The body loses blood. Injuries almost inevitably involve loss of blood, since tiny blood vessels are easily ruptured. The escaping blood seeps between layers of body tissue and is further distributed by the effects of gravity. This can explain why a bruise is not always on the painful part. If a significant portion of circulating blood is lost, this can cause a major disturbance in blood pressure, often more serious than the initial injury. Bleeding should always be staunched, (taking care with a puncture wound, for foreign bodies) with cold water, pressure and elevation rather than a 'tourniquet'.

Soon after injury has occurred, the small vessels begin to constrict and the blood clots. This is achieved by the coagulating cells in the blood, the platelets, which together with the *fibroblasts* or *matrix cells*, link body tissue back together again. Providing an injury is not aggravated, all this happens quite quickly so it is wise not to move an injured person unnecessarily, unless they are in a position of greater danger.

There is inflammation and pain. Simultaneous with blood loss is the action of the undamaged structures nearby, which encour-age adjacent vessels to dilate and allow blood which is more fluid than usual to arrive at the injury. This blood contains an increased number of white blood cells, *leucocytes* which scavenge the injury, and is termed exudate. The exudate is very effective in disinfecting the injury, helping to stiffen the area and inhibit movement which would complicate the damage. Its presence also stimulates the growth of new tissue.

Heat, redness, swelling and tenderness all indicate exuda-tion. Considering what value there is in such a spontaneous response, these secondary pains should be borne bravely but massage intervention can alleviate much of the dis-comfort. Treatment of an injury begins with pain control, and careful management aims to prevent complications from misinterpretation of reactions.

COMMON INJURIES

Where possible it is preferable to deliver a seriously injured person to the nearest medical services. This is necessary so that all aspects of an injury may be examined properly. You might be called upon to adminster first aid, but more likely your partner will be consulting you *after* diagnosis. The treatment described here assumes a competent diagnosis has been made; if you are ever in the position of handling an injury without medical assistance, you must trust in your own abilities, follow the principles of first aid and proceed with a confidence which will reassure the injured.

Dislocation

This usually means that a joint has been forced from its normal position, and relocations are done by experts often under general anaesthetic. I was once a member of a team of five 'non-experts' who successfully relocated a dislocated shoulder on a remote island, by candlelight. We may have been helped in that the injured party was also suffering from an excess of alcohol; certainly the collective 'shock' of the team which made the decision to risk the procedure felt greater than his!

Injuries to Bones

These are often masked by severe joint injuries. The most serious bone injury is a *fracture*, which is usually so obvious and limiting it is hard to imagine the not uncommon circumstance of some walking around unaware of their broken leg. Fractures range from this very simple 'stress' type to very complicated situations where bone fragments interfere with other tissues (such as a rib with a lung). Perhaps because of the confidence we have in the bones' mending, other factors such as sprain and rupture which are associated with fracture, are neglected; massage treatments are indicated both during and after the immobilization of fractures.

Injuries to the Spine

These are most likely to take place at recognizable stress points between specialized vertebrae: for instance, from neck (*cervical*) to chest (*thoracic*), and at the junction of the spine and pelvis (*sacro-iliac*). More serious spinal injury involves unacceptable pressure on the *discs* between the vertebrae, which act as shock absorbers. The discs are designed and accustomed to the varying pressures of posture and are reduced in thickness as the day progresses – like cushions on furniture – recovering their shape with rest. With uneven pressure, however, the disc can be squeezed on to adjacent structures such as a spinal nerve ('trapped nerve'), and the local and radiating pain can be intense.

Fractures of the spine are medical emergencies.

Aligned posture rather than exercise is the key to maintaining improvement of spinal problems; but the reasons for better posture have to be attractive and more fun for your partner if good massage work on the spine is to be lasting. Using your knowledge of the skeleton, you might be able to demonstrate:

- that their spine is central to their body (more than it is their 'back') and is designed to make standing up effortless;
- that greater attention to holding on to the muscles of the abdomen (even with their hands!) is more important than trying to relax a tight back (Figure 45);
- that sitting down produces *more* strain on an aching spine than standing upright;
- that gentle walking or lying down with the legs raised and flexed, although extremes, are equally relaxing for the spine.

Injuries in Sport and Leisure

These are experienced because of unfitness, faulty technique and over-enthusiasm. All sports carry a greater risk of injury than everyday life, especially when they are done to offset an 'unhealthy' lifestyle. Sport can make one-sided demands on the body, and stresses in competitive sports sometimes override the benefits of training.

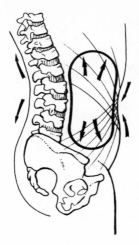

Fig. 45   How muscles of the abdomen support the spine

Rehabilitation

In the form of special exercises, this plays an integral part in massage where the muscles' helpers, the *ligaments*, which support the joints, are also damaged.

Injuries to Joints

These usually occur from falls, and range from sprain, where the ligaments are stretched or torn, to dislocation, a serious and violent loss of posture. Often a joint will accept injury to spare fracture of a main bone. This may be expedient in the short term, but joint injuries heal slowly and can have later rheumatic-type difficulties if treated badly, whereas bones almost look after themselves.

Joints are tolerant of slower, extreme pressures while light, jerky movements can easily stretch them. Manipulation techniques make use of this 'quick-snap' principle for therapeutic purposes where joints have become fixated. If you have experienced this form of treatment on your spine, you will recall how your conscious attention is often diverted by your practitioner's conversation; for instance, 'Do you know how many osteopaths practise in Arkansas?' – and as you search for a meaningful reply, your troublesome joint is thrust back into alignment.

Strong, supple muscles are the best protection against joint injuries. Torn ligaments can be repaired surgically, but provided the torn parts are in contact and remain still, healing will occur spontaneously. It has been shown that even a severed Achilles tendon (above the heel) recovers if the parts are simply set against each other.

Injuries to the Skin

These include abrasions, lacerations, burns and scalds. All these injuries respond favourably to the application of hydro-therapy. The skin has three layers: the *epidermis, dermis* and *subcutis* (Figure 46). It is extremely regenerative and you will have noticed that superficial scratches to the epidermis often recover completely within forty-eight hours. For deeper wounds, water treatment provides the ideal conditions for effective pain relief, cleansing and protection.

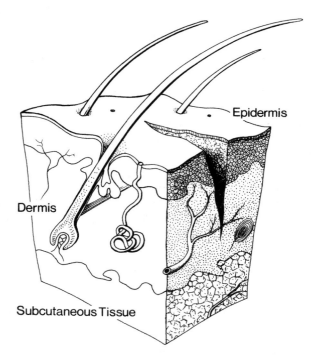

Fig. 46

Burns which penetrate the skin or cover a major portion of its surface require complex medical attention because of the skin's important organic functions, but even then moisture is regarded as helpful aid.

Another obvious benefit from using hydrotherapy on the skin is that stitching may be avoided, save in dire circumstances, and deeper cleansing is possible, which discourages scarring.

Injuries to Muscles and Tendons

These include tears, ruptures and strains. Muscles protect as well as move the body, and are called upon to make heroic rescues. Muscle tissue receives extraordinary energy at times of danger, but our underlying level of fitness will determine our speed of reaction. Certain sports and occupations, however, call for development of one set of muscles beyond others, and many injuries result from this imbalance.

Serious muscle injury requires complete rest, and if we find it hard to resist moving, we can end up in a 'plaster cast'. Though effective as a prison and punishment, this is not necessarily helpful to the injury, which tends to get isolated from the body to which it rightfully belongs.

Recurring injuries in fit people suggest an inappropriate choice of sport, and within teams people have to be careful to play in positions which suit their physique. To gain experience of injury, massagers could attach themselves as general therapists to sportspeople. I know of a new practitioner who has offered his services to a local American Football team (a sport fairly new in the UK), whose players anticipate injury as part of the game! With increased leisure facilities and emphasis on sport and health, increased demand for injury treatment is predicted.

TREATMENT FOR INJURIES

The management of an injury is comprised of three stages:

1. Limitation of its disturbance (24–48 hours).
2. Encouraging circulation; massage (after 48 hours).
3. Rehabilitation exercise (until normality restored).

I will describe treatment of an injured ankle.

Stage 1: Limitation of the Injury

This is achieved with compression bandages and cold water. The body's immediate reaction to injury is to produce exudate, the specialized blood which stimulates healing and cleanses the wound. It is important to restrict the amount of exudate by containing the injury from without; this discourages too much exudate forming and prevents stickiness around the injury which could give rise to adhesions. Adhering tissues create stiffness after healing and cause pain. They cannot be broken down later by massage and, if serious, will require surgery.

Another possible cause of adhesion is massage or exercise *too early* in the repair of an injury. Premature movement irritates damaged tissue and causes more exudate to form.

Use of the Compression Bandage

As soon as possible after the injury, the ankle should be surrounded with layers of cotton wool and a crepe bandage, with the wool interspersed between the turns of the bandage.

The injury should then be immersed or soaked in ice-cold water for 15 minutes (Figure 47). Cold helps relieve pain by reducing the conductivity of the nerves, and constricts the capillaries of the superficial structures to prevent further blood loss. For these reasons, *never* apply heat to an injury in the acute stage. Hot application is best used later to relieve muscle spasm and increase the blood supply to the injury.

The bandage is intended to hold the area in a firm support but with the structure in neutral, anatomical posture. Knees and elbows can be slightly flexed but ankle injuries fully flexed towards the knee. If possible, the injury should be placed higher than chest level. The bandage should be kept wet and cold.

At this point consideration can be given as to how to deliver the injured person to the medical services. Once diagnosis has been obtained, or if no services are available continue with stage 2.

Stage 2: Encouraging the Circulation

Within 36–48 hours, most soft tissue injuries have established healing reactions. Treatment now aims to encourage the

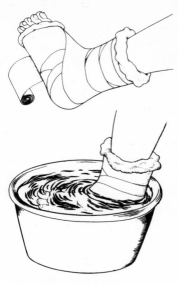

Fig. 47

circulation around the injury and keep the body comfortably at rest. The bandage is removed and the ankle inspected. (If there is no significant reduction of swelling, the bandage is replaced wet and cold for a further 24 hours.)

If the swelling has reduced but the injury is still painful use self-massage or contrast hydrotherapy.

Self-massage: Ask your partner to make active movements above and below the injury; in the case of the ankle, knee flexing and toe wriggling for two minutes. Avoid direct irritation and preferably have the leg raised. An infra-red (radiant) heat lamp can sometimes be used at this stage.

Contrast Hydrotherapy: Apply a very hot towel alternating with cold, 3 minutes each, 6 times, ending with cold. A spray of hot and cold water can be used instead, or for ankles or wrists, deep bowl immersions.

Note: If the injury includes a burn or cut, omit the hot application and alternate cold with 3 minutes rest.

Replace the compression bandage. A wet bandage should not be kept on overnight but the injury can be dry bandaged and kept cool by a surrounding wet towel. If painful during the night the ankle should be cold plunged but not dried before re-applying the bandage. The night bandage should be soaked off in the morning.

Massages

If, after 48 hours, the injury has improved to the extent that swelling and tenderness is reduced, you may begin gentle hand massage. If not, repeat stages above. Swelling that has not diminished indicates deeper damage, possibly to a bone or, not uncommonly, overuse by the injured. If your partner has experienced emotional shock as well as injury, these early stages can take a longer time to pass.

1. Repeat the hot and cold applications. Make strong effleurage up to (not over) the injury, then continue beyond. Repeat until there is further visible reduction in swelling.
2. Ask for some tentative movements around the injury for 2 minutes. Support the area with dry cotton wool and a crepe bandage and suggest your partner make normal use of their body, with rest periods throughout the day. The injury can be cold plunged when painful.
3. Two days later, if the swelling is further diminished: effleurage up to, then lightly over the ankle and firmly beyond. Friction stroke over the injury; circling with your finger tips, aiming to gently loosen rather than penetrate the skin. You may lightly oil your fingers with lavender blended essential oil, if your partner agrees. Repeat effleurage.

These strokes discourage the formation of adhesions from the circulatory response to the injury. They are not intended to disturb the healing process which is taking place in the new tissues. To assist in circulatory return, have the injury elevated or packed up on pillows during and after the massage.

Depending on the severity of the injury, massages can be continued every other day until your partner regains confidence in using the injured part. The dry bandage can be worn until the swelling disappears completely but should be removed overnight.

Stage 3: Rehabilitation

When near normal use of the injured part is achieved, an exercise programme is introduced after massage. (General body massage may be given after the first 24 hours of the injury. Apart from the relaxation benefits, particular attention can be given to areas which are compensating for the inconvenience of the injury – opposite leg, shoulders, and so on.)

Exercises have three aims: to improve strength, flexibility and co-ordination; and they have three styles: *passive, active* and *resistive.*

Strength

Passive: hold the foot carefully and move it around, reminding your partner of their ankle's movements.
Active: Ask your partner to move the ankle slowly and deliberately.
Resistive: hold the foot firmly. Ask your partner to move their ankle as before, trying (but not desperately) to overcome your resistance. Aim to balance out each other's tension, no one 'winning'.
Rest and repeat until fatigued (not the massager!).

Resistive movements are valuable in building confidence. They can convey to your partner, in a controlled way, how much their injury is improving. Strengthening exercises should be carried out on alternate days.

Flexibility

Passive: demonstrate stretching by pointing, flexing and twisting the foot, holding at extreme for 3 seconds.
Active: ask your partner to repeat the movements slowly.
Resistive: ask your partner to point the foot against your resistance; both agree to relax and immediately move the joint smoothly in the opposite direction to its comfortable limit.
Repeat flexing and twisting to both sides.

Injured tissues contract and lose tone while repairing. Stretches are introduced to regain elasticity and further improve circulation. Increased flexibility is not easy to measure unless you have known your partner's condition before injury. Comparison with non-injured sides of the body may guide you.

Co-ordination

Passive: walk backwards, sideways etc. Demonstrate the movement you are proposing. Go slowly and repeat if necessary.
Active: have your partner pass something (for instance, a ball), from foot to foot; play music and move in rhythm.
Resistive: ask your partner to stop in mid-step; change direction quickly as requested; balance on one leg, and so on.

Exercises in co-ordination help reintegrate an injury with the rest of the body. This involves a kind of reclaiming of a limb or posture by your partner, often an emotional experience. Be aware that you are encouraging rather than coercing, and constantly reassure.

Creativity with the exercise programme provides interest and stimulation for your partner's energy to recover. Injuries can involve emotional depression and oscillation between over-enthusiasm and despair. Your consistency in positively anticipating a satisfactory and realistic outcome to the injury is also vital.

Most injuries to the soft tissues (that is, the skin, muscles and ligaments of the joints of the limbs) can be treated along the lines of the above example. Trunk injuries are more complicated to manage due to greater nervous involvement. Injuries, like their owners, can be unpredictable, and you will develop tremendous patience as well as admiration while attending to your partner's healing processes. If you are in doubt about any aspect of a recovery, consult an experienced practitioner.

PREDISPOSITION TO INJURY

Our injuries possibly teach as more about ourselves than our illnesses do. The fact that recoveries are usually so complete distinguishes injuries from most disease processes. Having experienced injury, we learn how to avoid problems, whereas illness and the reasons we are given for its cause have relatively little effect on its incidence, if the major diseases of today are considered. (Ironically, the more we appreciate about modern disease factors, such as heart disease, the more they begin to sound like *self-inflicted injuries*.)

Recognizable factors associated with injury include: level of fitness, tiredness and 'tension', diet, and what we prefer to call 'accidents'.

Fitness

It is hard to find a definition of fitness with which everyone agrees. The condition of our lungs and heart are partly inherited; there are those who are advantaged by a better start in life, while others falter in spite of their healthy resolutions.

Although we are beginning to recognize activities which are potentially damaging, some people, not unreasonably, wonder just what we are preserving ourselves for, if not to enjoy a measure of indulgence! The attitude 'as fit as I need to be' may be more philosophical than complacent, and reflects the attitude of someone curled up, relaxed with a book and a cigarette, compared with a panting, defeated executive on an electronic cycling machine. A truly unfit person confidently knows what their limitations are.

Tiredness and 'Tension'

These can be two sides of the same coin, which suggests strain and pushing up to and beyond tolerable limits. Sometimes it would appear that tiredness is offered as a sign of commitment, yet there is no doubt that our reflexes and reactions are dulled by excessive tension.

Those who go unscathed from going 'all out' may succeed by making distinct changes in direction – work hard/play hard/ collapse/bounce back again. Effective, perhaps, but in ways other people find too demanding as a route to relaxation.

Diet

Malnourishment means poor growth and consequently poor repair. Affluent societies suffer not only from refined, impoverished food but from the complexity of a rich diet which takes as much energy to consume as it gives, and over-consumption of 'good' food can still result in a net loss in nutrition.

Perhaps the most researched and demonstrable dietary factory associated with injury is the way quasi-foods undermine body efficiency. Processed foods slow up healing, while fasting accelerates it; 'stimulating' foods deplete energy; popular weight-reducing diets contradict natural appetite.

Among the many controversies surrounding diet, confusion over fluid intake persists. Earlier recommendations to drink at least four litres per day have given way by fifty per cent but this is still at variance with present physiological knowledge; beyond a small amount, water requirements, like food, are relative to the individual's make up. There is evidence to show that a high intake of any fluid disturbs digestion and depletes strength. Body builders are careful to drink very little for days before a contest, which may serve as a clue to the injured.

Injuries as 'Accidents'

How would you define an accident? Are you able to find a definition which still makes you feel secure in the world? Perfectly trained, perfectly relaxed and perfectly nourished people incur injury, and when it happens we routinely call this an 'accident'. There is an assumption that accidents are unexpected, unavoidable and somehow unfair. For the majority of us this prospect does not prevent our wholehearted involvement in many intense, high-risk activities.

We are increasingly aware of the emotional investments in many illnesses. Do they also apply in the case of injuries? Perhaps not in the sense that being shipwrecked or present at an earthquake suggests the unavoidable nature of certain accidents. We do however hear accounts of the uncanny coincidences associated with such events.

'Accident prone', an expression hinting that we might have a tendency to fall into injury in relatively innocent circumstances, is a condition many will have experienced at some time in life. *What* gets injured at these times can be as intriguing as *why* it should have happened. If you are interested in reading further about injuries as accidents, read Karl Menninger's *Man Against Himself*, for fascinating, if often harrowing, accounts derived from his psychoanalytic practice. (This book is now out of print, so check with your local library.)

PREVENTION OF INJURIES

One positive way of facing the likelihood of injury might be to have regular modifications of the treatment which we know produces reliable healing as a preventative. This follows a traditional edict in natural therapy: 'The care is the cure and the cure is the care.'

This approach allows you to offer as part of your massages, emphasis on the containing, mobilizing and supportive elements of injury treatment. The methods are best learned on uninjured partners so as to have developed confidence for injuries when they arise.

Containment

The enforced rest of the massage session is the element equivalent to the use of a compression bandage: the body is immobilized, heat distributed and gravity offset. Many partners will become accustomed to the regularity of treatment but for someone who finds it easier to 'keep going than to stop', an enforced rest is unappealing; your massage strokes will have to justify your persuasion.

Less active partners will look forward to their treatment as a relief, and make their appointments well in to the future. While the former may follow your suggestion and take a holiday but be uncommunicative, the latter would send a postcard: a 'massage message'. For everyone, massage offers an interruption of what we become habituated to and helps us avoid some of the damage which otherwise it would be impossible to avoid.

Mobilizing

Our partner may not always appreciate our interest in the extremely tense areas of their body, since attention to a problem is not always as pleasant as a general treatment. However, as observers of what partners may be only vaguely aware of, we are obliged to attempt to free tension and unblock the circulation of the body. Great care is required to investigate deep tensions, as we have to avoid giving our partner the impression that they are in a worse state than they thought!

Your affinity with your partner's structure, and the personal rapport between you should allow you to introduce treatments which you consider would be helpful. (This is how practices mature, as partners come to rely on your feelings about their body as much as they do their own.)

Given the unexpectedness of injury, the mobilization movements of massage can be become a prophylactic part of your general treatments. Familiarization with the anatomy of joints will enable you to exercise the structures which strengthen them. Experiment and create your own rehabilitation programme. Very tired partners will be surprised to discover how stimulating the exercises can be.

Encouragement

Quite often emotional trauma can precede physical injury and, although I have described some injuries as 'trivial', we should take care not to minimize someone's feelings. Life's events affect people in unique ways and sometimes result in conflicting responses. Expressions of conflict such as grief and resentment are legitimate within treatment, leaving partners freer to respond, if, as practitioners, we are able to accept them.

Our challenge is not to immediately pacify but to let our partner interpret the strokes in a supportive atmosphere. Regular massages punctuate the hidden strains of life, and the knowledge that someone is maintaining an informed interest in our condition continues that support.

9

Self-Massage as First Aid

THERE MAY BE occasions when treatment is needed before you have the opportunity to contact a helpful friend or practitioner – emergencies rarely occur in ideal treatment conditions.

When your immediate need is to cope well with your situation until expert help is available, the following self-helps can be recommended. These procedures have been tried and tested in a variety of circumstances – on a desert island, in homes, and in high-tech hospital wards.

While primarily intended as first aid, you can use these coping strategies equally effectively as *preventatives*. By including them as part of health maintenance, it might be possible to avoid the build-up conditions which often precede an emergency.

When you have experienced first aids on yourself, I am sure that you will be confident to offer many of them to a friend in need – hopefully, not all in the same day!

GENERAL PREVENTION

A very obvious, though not widely adopted, way to minimize everyday strain is demonstrated by our domestic animals:

When it's not essential to stand up – sit down, with knees well flexed; if sitting is uncomfortable – lie down, with the spine curled.

Some might feel that circumstances and convention constrain

their attempts to follow this first aid. However, 'civilized' alternatives such as standing with the weight on one leg, sagging, or crossing one leg over the other from a chair are all token indications that the body is weary and is probably reflecting our feelings about the situation in which we find ourselves. It might improve a situation more than interrupt it if a brief resting posture can be found.

If it is truly impossible to relax more completely, and time is short, a useful, fleeting alternative to recumbence may be available:

1. Find a doorway with a surround deep enough to allow you to reach up and hold on (Figure 48). (In modern houses and offices it might be insufficient; sports shops sell a telescopic hand-hold which can be adjusted to fit a door space and you might be advised to invest in one as a consideration for both your body and the door.)
2. Hold tight but relax your arms straight. Let your arms bend slowly as you take up your weight through the arms.
3. Breathing out, imagine that you are sitting down on to a stool you can't quite reach. Let your knees bend naturally and keep your feet in contact with the floor.
4. As you feel your whole body stretching out, you can swing your knees gently from side to side, head slightly dropping forward.
5. When your grip begins to tire, draw your abdomen in firmly and put your weight back on to your feet and stand up slowly.

You can do this whenever you sense tension or tiredness in your body or in a situation, but later in the afternoon is the optimum time for many people.

FOR THE BACK

For no immediately apparent reasons, backs sometimes 'go'. There is usually a split-second awareness of something not quite right in our posture, followed by a seizing of all the muscles in the vicinity, if not the whole body!

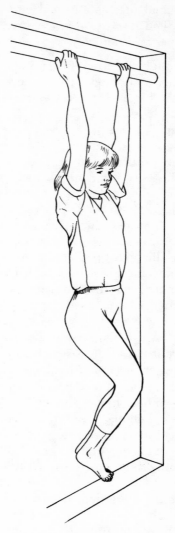

Fig. 48

Although essentially defensive in its reaction (the spine is safeguarded), the dramatic rise in muscular tension is very unnerving. Sometimes the body seems to 'freeze' and be incapable of any more movement at all without assistance, but for most people there is an overwhelming urge to relieve the weight from the spine.

Back emergencies are such universal experiences that many

intuitive and original first aids have been developed. The following is suggested for any situation involving seizure of the lower and upper back muscles.

1. As soon as a problem arises (for instance, from lifting, twisting, falling, and so on), place the body weight forwards, on to the hands; lean on to furniture, or if severe, get down on all fours.
2. Breathe as deeply as possible (oxygen helps relieve spasm) and try to assess the sensation. It is very likely that one side of the back is primarily affected and is involving other nearby muscles. Ask someone to look at your posture which will show obvious deviation to the primary tension. If alone, move gently to the left or right.
3. When you have decided which side has 'gone' (no need to worry about being absolutely right at this point), lie down on the edge of the body on that side and by degrees draw the opposite knee, up as high as possible to rest your weight upon. Let your elbow on the same side take the upper body weight and turn your head in that direction (Figure 49).
4. Keep the other arm on the opposite side of your body. This should allow you to breathe deeply again and you can check if your back feels easier. (If you have mistaken the side of greater tension, the above will be extremely uncomfortable, though not damaging, and you can slowly and reliably turn over to the correct side.)
5. Rest for a few minutes, reassuring your back muscles by a. carrying out regular, deep, controlled contractions of your abdomen, and b. imagining the whole of your trunk being compressed towards the earth by the force of gravity.
6. If feeling easier, gingerly return to the all-fours position. Try to straighten your spine to an upright position by climbing up a piece of furniture, but stay on your knees. If another spasm occurs, return to the former position for a few more minutes.
7. Trying again, make your way to seek assistance, preferably on your hands and knees, and then wait in the former horizontal position.

Don't feel defeated if this procedure is not immediately successful; you will probably have reduced your pain and

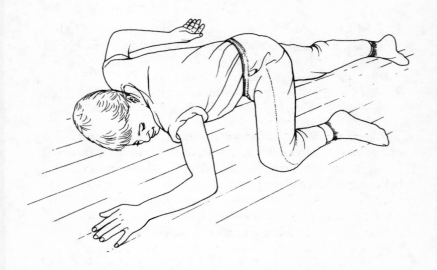

Fig. 49

certainly have minimized the work your practitioner will need to do with you.

You may recognize the horizontal position as very similar to the 'recovery' position of conventional first aid, and mothers may remember it as a relief from pressure on the growing abdomen.

Rehearse the sequence now if you have recurring back problems.

FOR A BLOW TO THE BODY/EMOTIONAL SHOCK

Both experiences are very similarly recorded by our system, and the first aid is common in both circumstances: *containment*.

People who have received upsetting news often speak of the impact in physical terms – 'It nearly knocked me over.'

The physiology of reaction has been described in detail in the chapter on 'Injuries', and the response to emotional upset also affects the circulatory system of the body.

For a Physical Blow, Fall, etc.

1. Assuming there is no bleeding, seize the injured part in both hands, if available, and compress it as firmly as possible for 3 minutes. If bleeding, apply a pad first, and if glass is in the cut, compress *around*.
2. Bind with a cold cloth, avoid weight bearing, and if pain lasts more than 12 hours seek advice.

This is an obvious treatment for a sprain, minimizing swelling and pain. Avoid moving the area until comfortable, otherwise a more serious condition could develop. Massage above and below, and breathe deeply.

For Emotional Shock

1. Find a soft place, lie down, and slightly curl up. Hold yourself by folding your arms around the chest and abdomen. Do not 'squeeze' as you need to be able to breathe easily.
2. Occasionally relax your arms and move your toes and fingers for a few seconds. Repeat until you feel more comfortable.

Self-applied 'containing' pressures imitate the exudate property of the blood for internal injury: reassuring immobility. This reduces the fear which always accompanies 'shock' and we are more easily able to move into the second stage of reaction – the increase of circulation, which gets us gently moving again.

FOR THE NECK

Problems with our neck muscles can be very psychological (the Bible speaks of stiff-necked people) but the neck, although exquisitely designed, is a vulnerable structure: heels on our

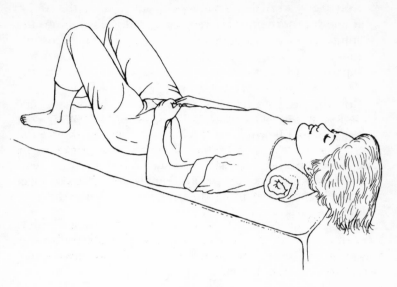

Fig. 50

shoes cause the head to tilt backwards and shorten the neck; most of us hear better from one ear and consequently twist the neck around to the clearer side; violent movements such as car collisions, while sparing the vertebrae, may tear at the neck's delicate nerves and blood vessels. This in turn may lead to referred pains in the arms.

The joints of the neck are normally very flexible but when continually misaligned, compensatory tensions build up around the bones (often heard as 'crackling' during neck exercises). The neck may eventually have to be manipulated and exercises followed to restore posture.

If you would like to encourage a relaxed centredness of your neck try this:

1. Roll up a small towel to make a diameter of approximately 3 inches.
2. Lie flat on your back with your feet drawn up to stand near the buttocks.
3. Place the towel under your neck, not your head, so that the normal inward curvature fits neatly over the towel (Figure 50). Relax your jaw.

4. Roll the head slightly from side to side against the towel.
   If one side of the neck feels tighter, roll the head into the
   stiffness for a few seconds, then slowly roll as far as possible
   in the opposite direction. Rest. Your neck should feel
   supported while the tight muscles stretch lightly. Breathe
   deeply and relax the jaw again.
5. Roll the head slowly back to the centre; lie on one side
   and push with your arms to become upright. Move your
   head around lightly.

Discomfort in the face and eyes benefit from this treatment. For sinus-type congestion, apply a hot cloth over
the cheeks, and a cold cloth to the feet during the procedure.

FOR THE ABDOMEN

Pains in the abdomen can mean something very serious since
our organs are normally relatively insensitive (Gandhi, the
founder of modern India, is reputed to have had his appendix
removed without anaesthetic). Before we can assume anything
dire, however, we should consider that acute abdominal discomfort is usually the result of indigestion.

Two common causes are eating foods together which
can be incompatible, such as fats and starches, and eating when anxious, thereby lacking the necessary digestive
juices.

The pressure which builds up in the intestines from these
conditions may be substantial but can be relieved. I was able to
congratulate someone on the spontaneous discovery of this first
aid. He was a driven, anxious person who ate like a carnivore,
and usually on the run: 'I regularly got a pain in my abdomen
and I always felt I should press on it. One day I did and it
went away. It doesn't happen so often now but the pressing
still works.'

1. Lie down with knees bent up. The area around your
   pain may feel hard. Rub gently with the heel of your
   hand.

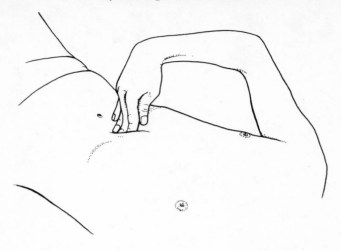

Fig. 51

2. Increase the pressure until you feel your abdomen softening. Find the painful spot with your fingertips and slowly begin to press through as if towards the spine (Figure 51).
3. You may detect a release or gurgle and increased relaxation of the abdomen. Rub again in a clockwise direction.
4. Draw your knees up towards your chest and hold on with your hands. Relax and breathe deeply.

Reflux (acid) from the stomach back to the mouth might suggest the beginning of conditions in the upper digestive system which you should consult your practitioner about.

FOR CONSTIPATION

We might chew well when we are upset, but our intestines function erratically. Constipation means a retaining tension in the large intestine and is often associated with conflict between personal and social life.

The condition is not in itself a disease but is thought to be a precursor to some diseases. It is not always an uncomfortable

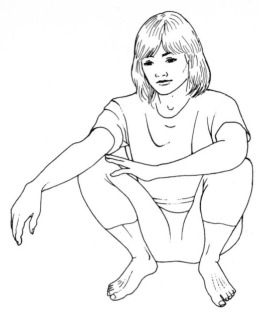

Fig. 52

experience although we may feel under obligation to conform to the eliminative 'norm' of a daily bowel action. It is this valiant effort that can produce the unnecessary distress.

1. Practise squatting by holding on to a friend or door handle and lowering your hips between your feet. Try to keep the feet flat.
2. Relax your neck forwards and practise retracting your abdomen, holding back for a few seconds at a time (Figure 52).
3. When you have suppled your hips, proceed to the toilet seat. Squat on the unit as you have been practising. If you can't manage this without fear of falling, sit down and raise your feet on a box so that your knees are higher than your hips.
4. Retract and slowly release your abdomen a few times.
5. Make a fist and massage deeply around your abdomen, especially on the left side.
6. Relax and breathe deeply. Avoid bearing down, and don't try to empty the bowel which should be an unconscious

action. After a few minutes, success or not, get up. Repeat the procedure throughout the day if necessary.

Consult a practitioner about recurring abdominal problems which do not respond to first aids.

FOR MENSTRUAL PAINS

More than the elimination involved in the period itself, the change in lower back posture which accompanies it is potentially hazardous. Ligaments in the pelvis release their control, lower back curve increases as the abdomen distends and becomes congested.

Contrary to some views which would have women do no physical activity at this time, many of the discomforts of menstruation can be relieved by simply inverting the pelvis. This lessens gravity's magnification of symptoms and is pleasantly relaxing for the abdomen and legs, which also become pressurized.

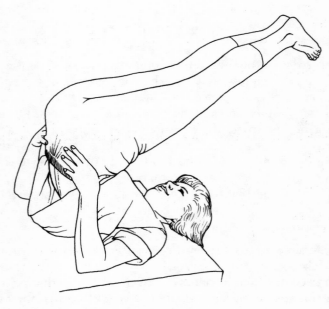

Fig. 53

1. Lie down with your knees slightly bent. Roll up on to your shoulders and using your elbows as props, support your hips with open hands (Figure 53).
2. When steady, move your legs around slowly and rotate your ankles, flex your toes and so on.
3. Breathe slowly and observe your abdomen go in and out as you breathe.
4. Remain in the position as long as comfortable, for a maximum of 1 minute. Recover very gradually, avoiding bumping on your spine and pelvis, by bracing your hands against the floor as you roll down.
5. When your spine is flat on the ground, hug your knees to your chest for 10 seconds.
6. Don't get up straight away; you could follow this with light abdominal massage.

I include this first aid on the recommendation of female colleagues. It can be done before, during and after the period; consider this an important time to take care of your posture. If you are unsure about how to invert your body, consult a Yoga teacher.

FOR THE EYES

In everyday life our eyes tend to dominate our other senses; we even use the expression 'I see' when understanding something not necessarily connected with looking.

Increased pressures on the eyes cause them to sting, blur and ache; internally the eyes are very responsive to changes in nervous energy and the emotions. In spite of this, their powers of recovery are acute and they do not appear to suffer from overuse (except in monotonous gaze and focusing).

This first aid, called 'Palming', rests the eyes and relaxes the neck muscles which are concerned with their effective circulation.

1. Sit close to a table and loosen the clothes from around your neck.
2. Place your palms (not fingers) over the eyes so that no light can enter. Lean forward and rest your elbows on the table (Figure 54).

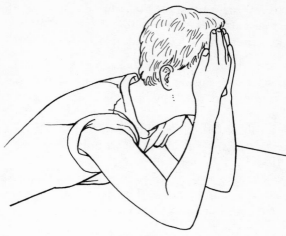

Fig. 54

3. Your hands should almost completely support your head. (Notice how tense the neck muscles become when you lift your head back slightly.) Let your face sink into your hands.
4. Have a mental picture of a vivid, colourful scene, with changing perspectives; 'look' with your physical eyes, exercising your eyes as if the image was outside your body.
5. After 1 minute, let the image fade, and relax your eyes into the darkness of your palms. Breathe deeply 6 times.
6. With eyes closed, slowly sit up straight and 'wash' your face with your hands, drawing away from the centre to the sides of the face. Open your eyes gradually.

If you are concerned about your eyes for any reason, do this twice a day and have neck massage.

FOR THE FEET

Our feet are confined almost from birth in a way that no other part of our body would accept. This is not always for protection and, by the time we realize this, irreversible compensations may have taken place – fallen arches and toe deviations to name the most common. It seems a pity to deny the feet their place in an otherwise relaxed body, and free-moving feet are themselves a great assistance to other disorders (for example, simple foot exercises in heart disease).

Choose from this selection of 'feet firsts' or do them all.

1. Take off your shoes and socks. Creep the feet forwards and backwards using clawing actions of the toes; rise up on tiptoe; curl the toes back as far as possible and hold till aching.
2. Put a rubber ball under the foot and roll it backwards and forwards along the instep. Run ankle-deep water in the bath and paddle for 3 minutes.
3. Play a cold shower as strongly as you can bear on the soles of each foot and against the calves for 2 minutes. Don't dry the feet but wrap them in a towel and lie down with your legs raised.

These aids also sometimes help with headaches. The water sessions are also useful when you are feeling low or just getting back on your feet after illness.

FOR THE NIGHT

Sleeplessness, while disturbing, is not regarded as fatal and if we can't get off to sleep or stay asleep we need to develop the the same philosophical view as the constipated. Sleeping is not something we do but rather comes over us; often the real complaint is being awake to ourselves, our thoughts and sensations best forgotten for a time. There is also the irony that for some who do eventually get off to sleep, they are unable to wake clearly in the morning.

This aid is another form of Hydrotherapy.

1. Be ready for bed and go to the wash basin.
2. Run cold tap water over your hands and forearms until they are chilled but not numb.
3. Do not dry your arms but mop your skin and go straight to bed.
4. Adopt your chosen sleeping position (preferably curled up) and put your hands between your arms and chest.
5. Forget your desire to sleep, and lie still, breathing deeply . . . goodnight . . . insomnia isn't worth losing sleep over . . .

10

'Massage!' Taking it Further

O F ALL THE therapies introduced to me as a student naturo-
pathic practitioner, therapeutic touching was the most
revolutionary. Up until then I had only experienced the
cool detachment of the family doctor, and I associated the
physiotherapies with infirmity. I subsequently learned that
this had not always been so in healthcare, and today among
my favourite written resources are massage textbooks published
at the turn of the century.

During my studies in Edindurgh I came across an article
in the London *Sunday Times* from the 1970s which reported
on the extent of physical contact between adults throughout
the world. Figure diagrams, shaded red for contact, blue for
little or none, showed that the further the distance from the
equator the less contact occurred. In Scotland, the blue was
only relieved by a token smattering of red on hands, head
and genitals!

I tried to reconcile these findings with positive response of
patients to massage at the clinic. Everyone seemed to look
forward to their treatment and regretted that this would be
what they missed most on their return home. For many reasons but perhaps most importantly, accessibility, therapeutic
massage was hard to find. Formerly, professional practitioners
were indeed few and far between; today the practice of massage
is enjoying a well-deserved revival among everyone who is
enthusiastic to live a healthy life.

However, because of the associations between massage and
prostitution, because massage continues to be confused with
physiotherapy, and because it is almost easier to admit to

having migraine than massage in our culture, there are still some problems to be overcome. I will discuss some of the issues which come up for people attending introductory massage courses with their friends and family, and describe professional training opportunities for those wishing to make a serious study of massage.

PRACTICE

For many enthusiasts, lack of practice hinders the development of their massage. Curiously, for new massagers, friends seem to prefer paying a stranger for something which is being offered freely. This is something to be overcome since it can perpetuate the idea that massage is an exclusive profession, done only by experts.

A genuine inhibition for friends and acquaintances arises from the conflict between intimacy and detachment. For good reasons, professionals tend not to treat their spouses, not that there need be any practical difficulty; what is unexpected is the paradoxical detachment *and* intimacy of massage.

Because a massage partner is not relaxing with you but *through* you, it can be alarming for your intimates to be aware of an unusual distance developing. For this reason, when partners are being chosen in the early sessions of a massage course, it is important that there must be freedom to reject a partnership offered, without an individual feeling this as a negative rejection – it can be that someone feels too *strong* an attraction rather than the opposite.

For a non-professional attempting to build up a practice, bartering may be the best way. If someone has something which you feel is a good trade for your treatment, make a clear offer. On talking over a particular problem someone may be having in getting practice, we often find that rather than friends' reticence to be massaged (most are willing to a degree), the answer lies in the clarity of the massager's approach.

CONFRONTATION OR ENCOUNTER?

A major problem to be encountered sooner or later in practice, is how we reconcile our sexuality with the physicality of massage. This is not a unique problem since research has suggested that the subject of sex occupies much adult thinking time.

Sexual issues can arise in all human encounters, and quite naturally we have come to terms with them in reality of a treatment session. Just as in other life situations, the beginning of clearing away any sexual ambiguity in massage starts with the awareness of our own individual sexual consciousness. If this consciousness is a little dormant, you can be sure that it will awaken as your interest in massage grows. This can come as a shock to promising massagers, and misinterpretation may cause a retreat; even if you consider your attitude already enlightened, you will find that it is soon put to the test.

It is not always possible to know when a personal encounter is becoming sexualized. Many sexual responses take place at 'sub-conscious' levels, and while your massages are intended to be pleasurable experiences, you may never know the quality of the sensation your partner is experiencing. From the point of view of this book, however, although the whole of a person's body may be regarded as 'sexual', the reproductive organs are not included in massage. (Gynaecologists and urologists, experts who specialize in this area of treatment, usually require their subjects to be anaesthetized . . .)

In a class discussion group, many women massagers said they felt comfortable about sexuality being part of the massage experience. One man agreed, but when asked if this would include his male partners, he wasn't so sure. Some women in the group felt that the 'problem' could be minimized by only working with partners of their own sex.

While it is very important to feel comfortable with your partner, in your early practice it may not be helpful to exclude people because of gender; massage offers an opportunity of honestly addressing sexuality, and your partner's embarrassment or naivety may only be mirroring your own. Sexual expression can also be representative – of anger, fear and other distress – and your honest attitude is just as important as your skill and attention in treatments.

Good massage engages the sensual aspect of our sexuality

although this is not necessarily clear for first-time partners. People who are well controlled in daily life can be surprised at the depth of gentle massage; some may interpret new sensations as alarming, feeling the movement of their tensions as more chaotic than relaxing. From their position, a partner may find it hard not to feel that you are provoking these changes rather than facilitating them.

It is the sensual element which forms the basis of unspoken rapport in massage, and for experienced practitioners it is an important aspect of the therapeutic relationship. Contemplate that your partner, usually being less experienced than you are, generally responds according to your way of treating. The language may have been intended to be transcendental but we all laughed when, breaking the silence of a beginner's course, a partner exclaimed, 'This is beyond sex!'

PROFESSIONALISM

If you have relieved someone's headache by massage, you are likely to attribute this to the methods you have used, which will have lessened the tension in the neck muscles. If you are using massage to help someone cope with a condition which has been acutely diagnosed, such as asthma or hypertension, you are more likely to be deploying massage's general effects of relaxation and reassurance.

The beneficial massages which have been described in this book, while undoubtably therapeutic, are available to most beginners. Many people, with the briefest of training have shown a natural capacity to massage.

Physiotherapists need special training because their career directs them towards medical conditions and complications outside the scope of this book. In contrast, everyday massage aims to help prevent medical problems arising.

In your early practice, massage itself allows you to 'learn as you go', but at some point your successes will begin to activate your real curiosity about what's really going on – this is when you may feel like pursuing a professional course. There are many approaches to a formal study of massage although not all, surprisingly, emphasize the humanistic element.

FORMAL TRAINING

A professional course will involve *examination*, and the more 'natural' massagers find this an unappealing prospect. In order to achieve accreditation, however, it is generally accepted that a student should be able to favourably impress an examiner, who acts as a representative on behalf of future 'clients'. At this stage the practitioner should be able to show style in handling rather than expertise, and be able to articulate the rationale for the treatment and the explanation of its effects.

Many serious massage students are those looking for a change in career or, more often, mature people who have sensed that in spite of having no clinical background, massage is just 'right' for them. Increasingly, however, established professionals from the health field, such as nurses, home visitors, and remedial teachers are finding that they can incorporate supportive massage into their work.

There are many independent schools of massage offering a wide variety of depth in method of study. Tutorials usually take place at weekends, allowing part-time attendance for practical coaching and guidance on study and learning methods.

Some courses are self-examined, where tutors assess the student on the technique or school of thought which they uphold; others are linked into wider professional organizations.

The Independent Examination Council (ITEC) combines both methods, offering a modulated examination system, where practitioners can move through basic massage therapy to aromatherapy, injuries, nutrition, reflexology, and sports exercise. This allows you to build up a practice gradually, offering general treatments from the beginning and adding to your expertise as you gain in experience.

The Northern Institute of Massage is a long-established organization which trains and validates practitioners in remedial forms of massage and manipulative therapies.

For readers wishing to practise massage outside the UK, I recommend the *International Massage & Bodywork Resource Guide*, published annually in the USA. This is a unique directory which lists schools, associations and laws relating to massage in ten different countries. (See p.115 for address.)

Some practitioners need guidance on the interactional

aspects of massage, and if this has not been covered to you satisfaction in training, your local university may offer a counselling course, or might advise on a trainer.

It is important to realize that your training course is merely the preliminary to the practice of massage. The word 'practice' is used within professions to make clear that a practitioner does not begin 'perfect' but uses work experience to develop, discover and refine their initial burst of enthusiasm.

When choosing a course, be aware of what is being offered or promised; you should expect clear instruction, access to your tutor's professional experience, and much encouragement to help organize your own plans, including post-graduate supervision.

Your school will be able to put you in contact with a professional organization for insurance purposes, but for most people the end of their course brings with it the feeling they are now *on their own*. This has to be, of course, and a practice grows from the individual effort, frustrations and sudden inspirations of the individual.

If for any reason you are unable to keep contact with your school or have no fellow practitioners nearby, make friends with other professionals, share problems and difficult cases with anyone you feel you can trust, and avoid at all costs the isolation which can occur in both the quietest and busiest of practices.

There is an attitude, even among 'alternative' schools that only trained professionals are competent to treat others, but as I hope to have indicated throughout the book, massage is a human rather than technical experience. It belongs to our senses, like the talent to cook a satisfying meal which does not poison our guests, or to be able to teach a friend to swim safely. If you decide, however, to formalize your interest in massage through a training course, I trust that your transition will be an integrated one – retaining the human touch while developing the responsibilities of professionalism.

In conclusion I offer every encouragement to you and your partners to follow the suggestions in this book; to be inspired to contribute to health and pleasure, and to continue to enjoy the giving and receiving of Massage.

CONTACTS

Up until now, UK law has allowed a lay person to practise a therapy freely and openly. However, in view of pending new European Community Directives, I strongly advise that you take formal examinations in massage if you wish to practise it as a career.

For a list of schools offering the ITEC examination system write to:

The International Therapy Examination Council
James House
Oakelbrook Mill
Newent
Gloucs GL15 1HD

For in-depth training contact;

The Northern Institute
100 Waterloo Road
Blackpool
Lancs FY4 1AW

The *Resource Guide* (See p.113) can be obtained from:

Noah Publishing
PO Box 1500
Davis
CA 95617–1500
USA

Appendix
Detailed Instructions for the
Muscle Diagram

- Get page 117 photocopied up to A3 size on card for stability: pages 118–19 can be copied up to A3 on coloured paper.
- Have scissors and glue to hand (solid paper adhesive is clean and fast drying).
- You may like to have some colouring pencils to distinguish the individual muscles.

The muscles have been numbered according to the order in which they should be stuck down on the skeleton. This corresponds to the way they appear to be layered around the body.

There are innumerable important muscles unrepresented, such as the supporters of the organs; and the ligaments which bind the joints are also omitted. With practice you will be able to detect all the muscles illustrated underneath your partner's skin. Studying the diagram will also encourage you to learn about muscle action and may help in identifying a deeper area of tension which you wish to treat.

'O' on the individual muscle indicates the origin or fixed point at which the muscle is anchored to the bone. This end should be stuck down on to the skeleton.

'I' on the muscle refers to the insertion point, attaching to the bone which it intends to move; leave it unstuck on the skeleton to suggest this.

You should be aware that the terms 'origin' and 'insertion'

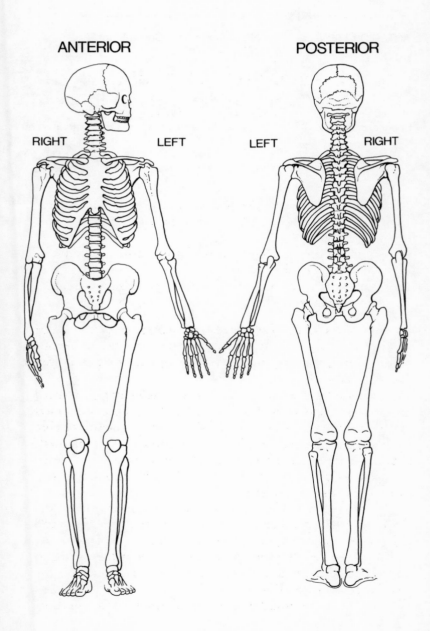

Massage

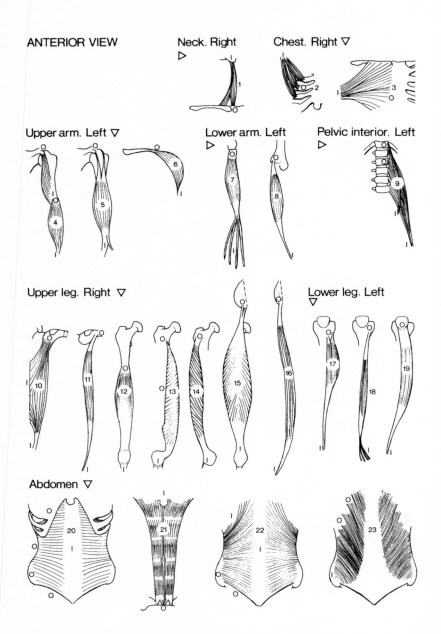

118

POSTERIOR VIEW

Back. Right ▽

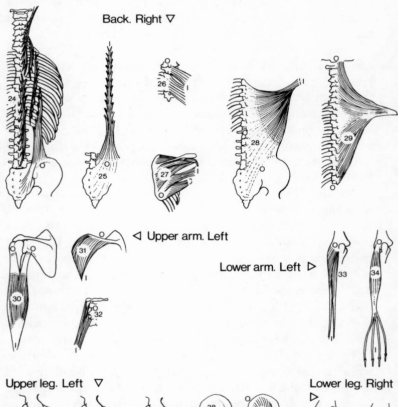

◁ Upper arm. Left

Lower arm. Left ▷

Upper leg. Left ▽

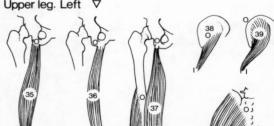

Lower leg. Right ▷

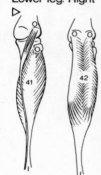

are relative, used for convenience by anatomists, who assume that the body is in a stationary, upright position for study.

For example, the broad back muscle (28. Latissimus Dorsi) 'originates' on the back of the chest and pelvis and 'inserts' on the upper arm so as to draw the arm close to the chest. (Ask a friend to stimulate this muscle by pinching the sides of your chest – you will immediately feel your arms clamp down towards their hands.)

However, from another posture the rules can change: if you can reach up and hold on to a horizontal bar above your head, try and draw your body upwards (chest towards arms); the origin and insertion principle will now be reversed. This is one of many anatomical paradoxes and you should begin to develop a philosophical approach from the beginning. For easy reference amongst colleagues, the origin of a muscle is regarded as the part nearest the spinal column; the point furthest away is the insertion.

Although we have been discussing independent action, in reality many muscles are involved in even the simplest movement. They co-ordinate to achieve the precision of poise and strength we take for granted in adult life. The main muscle which initiates a movement is given the title of 'prime mover', while its opposite neighbour, the 'antagonist', releases its tension slowly, which helps smoothness and control. (The Biceps and Triceps muscles of the upper arm are the most obvious example of this.) Other nearby muscles which co-operate to help align a movement are called 'synergists'.

To begin with, try laying a few muscles around the skeleton while tracing them on your partner's body; then build up a leg or arm or trunk section and begin to stick down the origins, lower numbers first. Notice that each origin has a piece of bone corresponding to its place on the skeleton.

ANTERIOR (FRONT) VIEW

Muscle of the Neck – right side

1. *Sterno-cleido-mastoid*: originates on the sternum and clavicle (cleido) and is inserted on a prominent part of the skull,

the mastoid. Cut out and stick along the clavicle (collar bone) and top of the sternum (breastbone).

Action: Independently, flexes the neck and rotates the head; together, the muscles cancel out each other's rotation, and flex the neck powerfully.

Drop your head forward and turn it to the side – you will feel the muscle working. We make a similar movement when lifting our head from the pillow to check the alarm clock – if we've overslept, the shock may send this muscle into spasm!

Muscles of the Chest – right side

2. *Pectoralis* (meaning 'breast'): *Pectoralis Minor* originates on the upper ribs and inserts on the scapula (shoulder-blade). Cut out and stick on to the ribs.
    Action: Helps fixate the scapula in shoulder movement.

3. *Pectoralis Major*: originates on both the clavicle and the sternum and inserts on the humerus (upper arm). Cut out and stick on to the clavicle and sternum.
    Action: Draws the humerus forward and rotates it inwards. This muscle gives shape to the upper chest and forms the front portion of the axilla (armpit); it is the main performer in the 'press up' exercise.

Muscles of the Arm – left side

4. *Coracobrachialis and Brachialis* (*brachium* means 'arm'): Coracobrachialis originates on the scapula and inserts on the humerus.
    Action : swings arm forward as in marching.
    Brachialis originates on the humerus and inserts on the ulna.
    Action: flexes the elbow. Cut out and stick on to the scapula and halfway down the humerus.

5. *Biceps* (originally meaning 'two heads'): originates on the scapula and inserts on the radius (smaller forearm bone). Cut out and place over muscle 4.
    Action: together, muscles 4 and 5 flex the arm at the elbow;

Biceps makes the familiar (though not exclusively) male bulge on the upper arm.

6. *Deltoid* (so-named after its Greek 'D' shape): originates on the clavicle and scapula, then converges to insert on the outside of the humerus. Cut out and stick on to the scapula.
    Action: abducts (draws away) the humerus from the side of the chest. The Deltoids are represented as epaulettes on military uniforms, signifying the wearer is strong and powerful.

Muscles of the Lower Arm

7. *Flexor Digitorum Profundus* (long flexor of the fingers): originates on the ulna and inserts on the terminal phalanges (finger bones). Cut out and stick on to the elbow.
    Action: flexes the last joint of the fingers. As an experiment in muscle control see if you can flex the fingers separately.

8. *Flexor Carpi Radialis*: originates on the humerus and inserts on the second and third meta-carpals (hand bones). Cut out and stick on to the elbow.
    Action: flexes and abducts wrist. When you hold a violin in place the wrist is controlled by this muscle.

Muscles of the Interior Pelvis

9. *Psoas Minor and Major* (pronounced 'Sohass'): originate on the last thoracic and all lumbar vertebrae; Minor inserts on the pelvis and Major on the femur (leg bone). Cut out and stick on to the spinal column.
    Action: Minor flexes the pelvis, i.e. tips it backwards; Major flexes the hip joint and rotates the femur inwards as in 'leg-crossing'.

Muscles of the Upper Leg – right side

10. *Gracilis* (meaning 'graceful'): originates on the pubic bone and inserts on the tibia (main lower leg bone). Cut out and stick on to the lower pelvis.

Action: adducts (draws inwards) the knee and helps flex it.

11. *Adductor Magnus*: originates on the ischium (lower pelvis) and inserts on the femur. Cut out and stick on to the pelvis.
Action: adducts (main adductor) the thigh. You may be uncomfortably aware of other adductors, not represented on the diagram, after you have ridden a horse or pillion-passengered for the first time!

12. *Vastus Internus* (large internal):
13. *Vastus Medialis* (large inside):
14. *Vastus Lateralis* (large outside): all originate on the femur and insert with Rectus Femoris via the patella on to the tibia. Cut out and stick on to the upper leg.
Action: help extend (straighten) the knee.

15. *Rectus Femoris* (upright thigh): originates from two points on the ileum (upper pelvis) and inserts together with the Vastus muscles on the tibia via the patella (kneecap).
Action: main extensor of the knee, plus flexor of the hip from its attachment to the pelvis.

Muscles 12–15 are also known collectively as the Quadriceps (four-headed muscle) because of their common insertion at the patella. Give a good follow-through kick of your leg to feel the full effect of the Quadriceps.

16. *Sartorius* (literally meaning 'tailor'): originating on the ileum and inserting on the tibia, Sartorius is the body's longest muscle. Cut out and stick on to the pelvis.
Action: flexes the hip and knee, and rotates the leg inwards. To sit like an old-fashioned tailor, use Sartorius to draw your knees outwards and sit cross-legged.

Muscles of the Lower Leg – left side

17. *Peroneus Longus* (*Peroneus* means 'boot'): originates on the fibula (smaller, outside bone) and inserts beneath the first metatarsal (foot bone). Cut out and stick on to the knee.

Action: everts (turns outwards) the foot and helps flex the ankle, as if to pull on a boot-lace.

18. *Extensor Digitorum Longus*: originates on the fibula and tibia and inserts on the last bones of the toes. Cut out and stick on to the knee.
Action: extends (uncurls) the toes and helps flex the ankle.

19. *Tibialis Anterior*: originates on the tibia and inserts on the underside of the first metatarsal and adjacent tarsal (ankle). Cut out and stick on to the knee.
Action: inverts (turns inwards) the foot and helps flex the ankle (like an inner boot-lace).

The ankle joint has many powerful ligaments (small fibrous bands) which protect the joint from over-stretching by its main muscles and from the weight of the body above. When the protection is overcome, the joint gives way and the ankle is 'sprained'.

Muscles of the Abdomen

20. *Abdominis Transversalis*: originates on the lumbar vertebrae, ileum and lower ribs, and is also attached to the lower back muscles. It encircles the abdomen and is inserted on the base of the sternum, and a central tendon running down from the chest to the pubis. Cut out and stick on to the pelvis and ribs on the *right* side only (so as to be able to observe the Psoas muscle on the left).
Action: constricts the abdominal contents like a 'corset'.

21. *Rectus Abdominis*: originates on the pubic bone and inserts on the fifth to seventh ribs. cut out and stick on to the pubis on the *right* side. (Remember that the right side of the skeleton is to *your left* as you look at it.)
Action: flexes the spine by pulling the chest forwards; assists Transversalis in containing the abdomen.

Inward contraction of the abdominal muscles produces successful evacuation of the large intestine (bowel). 'Bearing down' on the intestine encourages constipation by constricting its free action.

22. *Internal Oblique*: originates on the ileum, towards the pubis and also has attachments on the lower back muscles. It is inserted on the lower three or four ribs and the abdomen's central tendon. Cut out and stick on to the pelvis on the *right* side.

23. *External Oblique*: contrasts origin and insertion with the Internal Oblique – origin on the rib cage and insertion on the ileum. Cut out and stick on to the rib section of the Internal Oblique.
    Action: together, these muscles flex the trunk (forward); if the Internal, on one side flexes with the External of the opposite side, the trunk rotates, as when you sit up and turn to the side through one movement.

The Oblique muscles strive to retain a flattering shape to our waist often against considerable odds. Heroic exercises to regain abdominal musculature are often offset by unrestrained 'jaw' exercises – corrective movements taken to the point of strain only flatten the upper area and our organs are forced downwards, exaggerating the belly. The most advantageous abdominal exercises are achieved with the body inverted or semi-inverted (for example, the yoga Shoulderstand) while the legs are gently swung and flexed.

Having completed half of the diagram, you will be well acquainted with origins and insertions. You can now proceed to the next section, remembering that the body does not actually have a 'front' or 'back' but is really more cylindrical, with the spine at its centre.

Try to recognize which new muscles are 'antagonizing' the ones already stuck on by the description of their action. Later you could copy out the pages again and apply muscles to the front and back by pairs, as antagonists.

Another time, conceal the numbering and see if you can simply lay the muscles on the skeleton from memory.

Not everyone feels completely familiar with every muscle group even after considerable practical experience. If the whole diagram seems too complicated, take one group in an area you feel more confident about and let your curiosity lead you to other muscles in time.

POSTERIOR (BACK) VIEW

Muscles of the Back (spine and chest) – right side

24/25. *Sacrospinalis* (a collective term for erectors of the spine): all originate on the lower vertebral column and insert on the ribs higher up and eventually on the skull. Cut out 24 and stick completely on to the pelvis, spine and chest; stick 25 on to the sacrum (lowest spine).
Action: extends the spine and neck by drawing the vertebrae up on end. Sitting up from a slouch demonstrates Sacrospinalis.

26. *Rhomboid Minor and Major*: originate on the lowest cervical (neck) and upper thoracic (chest) vertebrae and insert on the edge of the scapula. Cut out and stick on to the vertebrae.
Action: rotate the scapula, drawing it towards the spine.

27. *The four scapular muscles in descending order:*
Supraspinatus: originates on the scapula above its spine (ridge) and inserts on the humerus.
Action: assists the Deltoid muscle in raising the arm.

Infraspinatus: originates beneath the ridge and inserts on the outside of the humerus.
Action: rotates the arm outwards.

Teres Minor: originates on the outer edge of the scapula and inserts on the outside of the humerus.
Action: assists Infraspinatus and helps keep the arm in the shoulder (ball in socket).

Teres Major: originates on the lower scapula and inserts on the inside of the humerus.
Action: rotates the arm inwards and helps retain the arm in the shoulder.

Cut out and stick the rib tab on to the chest so that the edge of the scapula lies adjacent to the Rhomboid muscles. You can then observe the spinal muscles by lifting the scapula.

28. *Latissimus Dorsi* (broad muscle of the back): originates on the sacrum, ileum and lower ribs and inserts to the inside of the humerus. Cut out and stick on to the spine and pelvis.
   Action: adducts (draws in) the arm, takes it backwards and rotates it inwards. The shape of this muscle creates the expanding 'V' shape to the back. Latissimus and scapular muscles form the rear portion of the axilla.

29. *Trapezius*: originates on the occipital (rear) bone of the skull and spinal column, down to the last thoracic vertebra and inserts on the ends of the clavicle and scapula. Cut out and stick on to the spine and skull.
   Action: elevates and draws back the shoulders as in 'shrugging'. You can detect Trapezius easily by pinching along the top of the shoulders.

Muscles of the Upper Arm – left

30. *Triceps* (originally meaning 'three heads'): originates on the scapula and humerus and inserts on the ulna (elbow). Cut out and stick on to the scapula.
   Action: extends the elbow in classic opposition to the Biceps muscle.

31. *Deltoid* (posterior view): see text at muscle 6. Cut out and stick on to the upper scapula.

32. *Levator Scapulae*: originates on the upper four cervical vertebrae and inserts on the top of the scapula. Cut out and stick on to the neck spine.
   Action: raises the scapula.

Muscles of the Lower Arm – left

33. *Extensor Carpi Radialis* (antagonist to Flexor Carpi 8): originates on the humerus and inserts on the base of the second and third metacarpal. Cut out and stick on to the elbow.
   Action: extends and abducts the wrist.

127

34. *Extensor Digitorum Communis* (antagonist to Flexor
    Digitorum Profundus 7): originates on the humerus and
    inserts on the terminal phalanges.
    Action: extends the fingers.

Clench and straighten your fingers to examine the perfectly
synchronized antagonism of the flexors and extensors. Notice
too how the muscles slim down from the arm to form slender
tendons (cords) which pass through the narrow wrist and into
the hand – this is extraordinarily intelligent since it prevents
the hands increasing in size from constant use as happens with
main muscle fibres.

Muscles of the Upper Leg – left

35. *Biceps Femoris*: originates on the ischium and inserts on
    the fibula and tibia. Cut out and stick on to the pelvis.
    Action: flexes the knee and rotates it outwards; extends
    (draws back) the hip joint.

36. *Semitendinosus*: originates on the ischium and inserts on
    the tibia. Cut out and stick on to the pelvis.
    Action: flexes the knee and rotates inwards; extends
    the hip joint.

37. *Semimembranosus*: originates on the ischium and inserts
    on the tibia. Cut out and stick on to the pelvis.
    Action: as Semitendinosus.
       Also illustrated on 37 is the second, shorter 'head' of
    Biceps Femoris which originates lower down on the femur.
    Cut through between the larger and smaller muscle and
    tuck the Femoris under and directly on to the bone to join
    its partner, leaving Semimembranosus as the uppermost
    muscle of the group.
       The flexing thigh muscles are commonly know as the
    'hamstrings' after the medieval punishment in which they
    were severed. They are often injured in sports activities
    and can take a considerable time to heal because of
    their involvement in upright posture and walking. Their
    insertions are easily found behind the knee.

38. *Gluteus Minimus*: originates on the outer ileum and inserts

on the outer part of the femur. Cut out and stick on to the ileum.

Action: abducts the femur and rotates it.

39. *Gluteus Medius*: originates on the rim of the ileum and inserts on the femur. Cut out and stick on to the ileum.
    Action: similar to Gluteus Minimus.

40. *Gluteus Maximus*: originates on the ileum, sacrum and coccyx (tailbone) and inserts on the femur. Cut out and stick on to the sacrum so as to observe Gluteus Minimus and Medius.
    Action: extends the hip joint and rotates the femur outwards as in an 'arabesque' dance posture.

The Gluteuls are vital in maintaining the upright posture of the body, and in conjunction with the hamstring and Quadricep group, walk the legs. Gravity also assists walking, allowing the femur to swing like a pendulum. Consciously relaxing the knee and ankle joints as the leg swings through for the next step reduces effort in the thigh muscles and is very useful when recovering from injuries to back muscles.

Muscles of the Lower Leg – right

41. *Soleus* (meaning 'like a fish'): originates on the tibia and fibula and inserts on the calcaneum (heel), the largest tarsal bone. Cut out and stick on to the back of the knee.
    Action: plantar (downward) flexes the ankle, i.e. points the foot.

The slender muscle also shown originating from the femur and inserting with Soleus is *Plantaris*, an accessory to the following muscle:

42. *Gastrocnemius*: originates on the femur and inserts on the calcaneum.
    Action: strong plantar flexor of the ankle, and because of its origin on the femur, it helps flex the knee.

Muscles 41 and 42 give force to our step when walking quickly or running; standing still, they raise the body on its toes.

For greater clarity have a section of the skeleton and muscle chart enlarged on the copier if you are especially intrigued by a particular part of the body.

You may have to repeat the positioning of the muscles until you are sure that you recognize the bony guidelines, so use your glue sparingly to be able to correct mistakes. Don't be deterred, however, since in the real body, muscle arrangement is not always as textbooks have described; for example, Psoas Minor, the slender internal muscle, is estimated to be absent in thirty per cent of the population!

Do let me have your comments on this way of learning about muscles.

Glossary of Terms Used in Massage

Abduct: anatomical term meaning to move (a limb) away from the middle line.

Adduct: opposite of the above: to move towards the middle.

Anatomy: the science of the shape and structure of the body and its parts. Initially daunting for serious massage students, they have the advantage of learning the living anatomy of partners as they learn to massage.

Artery: a tube-like vessel which carries blood away from the heart to the rest of the body. Arteries become progressively smaller, becoming *arterioles*, then minute *capillaries*, only one cell in diameter. Research has shown that stressful Western lifestyle can cause arteries to degenerate prematurely.

Arthritis: inflammation of the structures within a skeletal joint (*rheumatoid arthritis*). When the lining of the bones which form a joint become worn and painful this is called *osteo-arthritis*.

Autonomic Nervous System: explains how the involuntary or unconscious functions, like breathing and digestion are controlled. The ANS has two complementary aspects: *sympathetic* nerves, concerned with stimulating, energetic action (speeding up); and *parasympathetic* nerves, which inhibit (slow down). Through these mechanisms the body's internal environment is kept in harmony.

Bronchi: the branch-like windpipe which reaches into the lungs, continually subdividing in the manner of a tree. The smaller bronchi are called *bronchioles* and terminate in 'buds', *alveoli*, at which point the respiratory gases exchange. While the 'trees' of our lungs breathe out carbon dioxide, the trees on earth breathe it in; their out-breathing of oxygen is taken up by our lungs.

Bursa: fluid-filled pads which help protect the joints of the limbs. When a joint is subjected to repeated, excessive pressures from without, the bursa may become inflamed: *bursitis*.

Biceps: a muscle which has two points of attachment to a bone (lit. 'two heads'), eg. the calf muscle, which can be felt behind the knee. Three points give *Triceps*, at the back of the upper arm: four points for *Quadriceps*, on the front of the thigh.

Caudal: towards the tail (of the spine).

Central Nervous System: the actions of the nerves of the body which comprise the brain, spinal cord and peripheries. The CNS is characterized as controlling the conscious and deliberate movements of muscle and mind. *Motor* nerves relay instructions to the muscles to contract: *sensor* nerves record pain, heat, cold, etc. for the brain's interpretation. Nerves exit from spaces between the joints of the vertebral column and can be adversely affected by disorders of the joint.

Cephalic: towards the head.

Circulatory System: the movement of the blood around the body via the heart and its vessels, arteries and veins, and the lymphatics.

Couch: a custom-built table for massage treatment. It may be fixed or portable and should be designed to the appropriate height for the practitioner. (To test: stand sideways by the couch, arms by your side; flex your wrist so that your palm is now horizontal – this is the recommended couch height for you.

Diagnosis: recognition of which disease a person has. Can lead to categorization and depersonalization of the patient/client. Some physicians prefer to ask: 'Which type of person has this disease?'

Diaphragm: the dome-like muscle which separates the contents of the chest from the abdomen. The diaphragm's active function is to assist full working of the lungs, while rhythmically massaging the digestive organs.

Dermis: the true skin, lying just beneath the outermost protective layer. The skin retains delicate sensitivity while forming an effective waterproof and thermal barrier for the body.

Dorsal: towards the back.

Endocrine System: describes the influence of hormones on the body. Hormones are chemical messengers, concentrated in glands strategically placed around the body. At critical times in our development, hormones are released directly into the blood stream to bring about subtle changes in functioning.

Eversion: to turn outwards.

Fibrositis: inflammation of the covering of the muscles, arising from excess tension or injury.

G5: a mechanical massage appliance. It is hand-held and does not substitute but can complement hand massage. Also useful in treating injuries, the G5 has the basic design of a circular head of rubber which vibrates horizontally.

Hypertension: abnormal and undesirably high blood pressure. Can be evaluated subjectively or by the *sphygomanometer*, an inflatable cuff placed around the arm. Although the sphyg. translates simply to mean 'to measure the pressure', its appearance and mere attachment to the arm often significantly raises the blood pressure!

Hypotension: low blood pressure. Low blood pressure is not regarded as particularly unhealthy in the UK (although it is Germany, where hypotensives are medicated in the same manner as hypertensives in the UK). Lower than average blood pressure is accepted as less strenuous for the body, but higher-pressure personalities naturally question what the slower moving hypotensives are conserving themselves *for*!

Immobilization: placing the body in such a position so as to minimize strain, especially if injured. *Examples*: resting a flexed knee over a pillow; placing the arm in a sling.

Insertion: the end of a muscle which is attached to the bone it intends to move. *Example*: the main calf muscle *Gastrocnemius* inserts on to the heel bone and by pulling on it, points the foot.

Inversion: to turn outside in.

Kyphosis: derangement of the spinal column resulting in an exaggerated outward curve in the thoracic spine.

Lordosis: excessive inward curvature of the spinal column at the lumbar vertebrae.

Lymphatic System: a complementary circulation which parallels the venous return. Lymph, which is the water drained from tissues, together with disinfecting white blood cells, washes through from the peripheral body, cleansing and tidying *en route* back to the upper chest where it returns to the whole blood just before entry to the heart. The lymph is periodically drained as it passes through *nodes*, conveniently placed in crevices of the body: behind the knee, in the groin, under the arms, etc. The nodes also contain extra-powerful cleansing cells, *lymphocytes*, which can be transferred to the lymph in transit for emergencies of accident or illness.

Massage: manipulation of the soft tissues of the body for therapeutic purposes. Records of forms of massage have been recorded in all cultures from the earliest times.

Medial: towards the centre.

Partner: someone who agrees to be massaged or exchange massage.

Posture: efficient alignment of the skeleton relative to any position but usually associated with upright stance. Posture can also mean attitude, which suggests that positioning has emotional and physical components.

Practitioner: one who gives massage professionally or with a committed interest.

Prone: facing downwards.

Psychology: the study of thought, emotion and behaviour, distinct from *psychiatry*, which is a medical speciality which treats diseases of the 'mind'.

Quadriceps: see **Biceps**.

Reflex: involuntary contraction of a muscle resulting from an unexpected stimulus. Occurs as in the 'tickling' mistake of a massage stroke which is too sudden or deep.

Rheumatism: formerly used for general forms of arthritis.

Sciatica: inflammation of the sciatic nerve, which runs from the lower back, behind the leg all the way underneath the foot. Sciatica often accompanies disorders of the vertebrae when these are misaligned or compressed.

Scoliosis: lateral (sideways) deviation of the spine, which, viewed from behind, creates 'S' shaped curves. The three common spinal deviations described in the glossary may be *congenital* (since birth), or as a result of injury or adaptation to environment.

Slipped Disc: a misnomer for a pressurized intervertebral disc (usually lumbar). The disc, which is made up of a cushion-like material, cannot actually slip but sometimes protrudes and interferes with the nerves exiting the spine. Discs are not 'put back in' even by the most exotic techniques, but are released by support and gentle traction.

Specialist: a practitioner with a concentrated approach, usually well experienced but in danger of 'finding out more and more about less and less'.

Stress: an excessive, unrelieved cycle of tension. Distinct from *strain*, which is self-regulating (something is hurting and we usually 'stop'), stress may be harder to recognize subjectively.

Supine: facing upwards.

Tendon: the fibres at a muscle's end which attach it to a bone. Overuse of a muscle may inflame the tendon, producing *tendonitis*.

Therapy: literally 'to care for' and accompany a person in their illness. Parallel of *patient*, ('receptive to healing').

Tonus: slight, continuous contraction of muscles, which maintains posture and helps blood flow. Listening into tonus with our ear against the skin, we would hear crackling tensions, similar to sounds heard during head-rolling exercises.

Traction: lengthening of the spine, usually from external stretch. Spontaneous traction occurs throughout the spine on each exhalation.

Trauma: literally 'wound', having physical and psychological consequences.

Treatment: what the therapist offers: a 'treat'.

Triceps: See **Biceps**.

Vasoconstriction: diminution of the smaller arteries; pallor; the effect of cold water on the skin's blood vessels.

Vasodilatation: expansion of the smaller arteries; blushing; the effect of alcohol on the skin's blood vessels (we feel 'warm'). The rapidly alternating vasoconstriction and vasodilation of the abdomen's tiny blood vessels when we are nervous gives the sensation of 'butterflies'.

Vein: a tube-like vessel which conducts blood back to the heart. Relatively superficial, the veins can be seen and felt, especially when *varicose*, full of pressure and struggling to overcome the effects of gravity.

Recommended Reading

Amadon, A. *The Fold Out Atlas of the Human Body*, Bonanza Books, 1984.

Asimov, I. *The Human Body*, New American Library, 1963.

Bertherat, T. *The Body Has Its Reasons*, Heinemann, 1988.

Bettany, C. *The Thinking Body*, Arrow Books, 1989.

Curtis Shears, C. *Nutrition Science & Health Education*, Nutrition Science Institute, 1978.

Freud, S. *The Psychopathology of Everyday Life*, Penguin, 1975.

Hauser, G.B. *Better Eyes Without Glasses*, Faber, 1956.

Ingham, E. *Reflexology – Stories the Feet Can Tell*, Ingam Publishing Inc., 1984.

Knott, B.S. & Voss, E. *Proprioceptive Neuromuscular Technique*, Hoeber-Harper, 1962.

Lederman, E. *Good Health Through Natural Therapy*, Kogan Page, 1976.

Liechti, E. *Health Essentials: Shiatsu*, Element, 1992.

Lewis, S. *An Anatomical Wordbook*, Butterworth-Heinemann, 1990.

Li-Hui, J. & Zhao – Xiang, J. *Pointing Therapy*, Shandong Science Press, 1984.

Masters, P. *Osteopathy for Everyone*, Penguin, 1988.

Siegel, A. *Polarity Therapy*, Prism Press, 1987.

Thomson, C. L. *Hydrotherapy – Water and Nature Cure*, Kingston Publications, 1970.

Wildwood, C. *Health Essentials: Aromatherapy*, Element, 1992.

Wirhed, R. *Athletic Ability and the Anatomy of Motion*, Wolfe, 1984.

Index

kneading 25–6
Kneipp, Father 66

legs 19
 crossing 13–14
 massage 40–1
lemongrass 64
Ling, Henry 20–1

massage, approach 33
 formal training 112–14
 in China 1
 in Greece 1, 2
 in Hawaii 1
 in India 1
 in Rome 1, 2
 in the nineteenth century 2
 natural 3, 9–10
 setting 32–3
 when not to 33–4
Menninger, Karl 92
menstrual pains 105–6
mobilizing 50–4, 93–4
movement 6–7
muscles, function 11–13, 16–17
 injuries 85
muscle spasm 67

neck 14–15
 first aid 100-2
 massage 46–50
 mobilizing 53–4

oil 32–3
osteopathy 68–70

percussion 22, 26–7, 28
petrissage 22, 24–6, 28
Polarity Therapy 70–4
posture 12–14, 61, 82

reflexology 72–4

sage 65
scoop 45
sexual issues 111–12
shiatsu 74–7
shoulders, mobilizing 51–2
 shiatsu 75–6
skin 84–5
spinal reflexes 73–4
spine 12–13
 injuries 82
Stone, Randolph 71
strength 89
stretching 47–9
strokes 21–9
Swedish System 21
talc 32–3
tapotement 28
Taylor-Still, Andrew 68
tendons 85
tension 61, 91

varicosity 67–8

FOREWORD

This is an excellent resource of rich Scottish Verse, well written, to be enjoyed by both children and adults. It brings out our culture and language in an exciting way. I would strongly recommend that this Scottish resource be made available for all.

Gordon Buchanan
Headteacher, Southwood Primary, Glenrothes.

CONTENTS

WALKIN THE RAINBOW

COLOURFUL POEMS FOR COOL KIDS

JILL BENNETT
ELIZABETH CORDINER

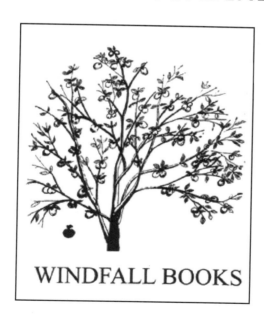

WINDFALL BOOKS

EDITED BY
LILLIAN KING

ACKNOWLEDGEMENT

Our sincere thanks to pupils and staff of Fife Primary
schools for the warmth and enthusiasm of their
welcome

The right of Jill Bennett and Elizabeth Cordiner
to be identified as authors of this work
has been asserted in accordance with the
Copyright, Designs and Patents Act 1988
A catalogue record for this book is available
from the British Library

© April 2008

Cover design - Belle Hammond
Illustrations - Belle Hammond

Typesetting, layout and design by Windfall Books
Published by Windfall Books, Kelty
01383 831076

windfallbooks@tiscali.co.uk
www.windfallbooks.co.uk

Printed by Stewarts Of Edinburgh

ISBN No: 978 0 9557264 1 5

ABOUT THE AUTHORS

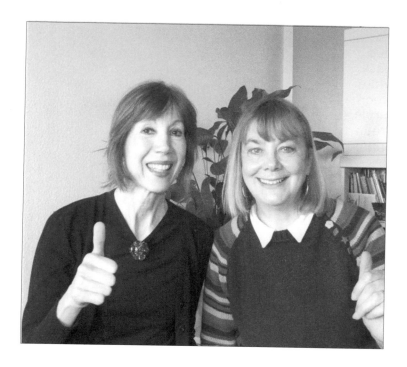

Elizabeth Cordiner, a retired Fife headteacher and writer from Glenrothes, has gone back into classrooms delivering Scots poetry to its natural and enthusiastic audience. All are having a rerr terr.

Jill Bennett, an ex school librarian, lives in Fife, and is a full time writer and tutor. This, her first collaboration on a poetry collection for children, arose out of the performances given in schools with Elizabeth. It was for both of them a joyful experience enriched by the delivery of the poems in the mither tongue.

What if colours had personalities,
just like people?
What if they could speak?
What would they say to you?
Hae a listen.

Imagine

If there were nae colours
That wid be like Irn withoot Bru
A bike withoot wheels
A bird withoot wings
A hert withoot love
Unimaginable

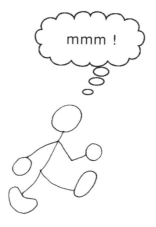

Rid

See me
Ah'm mad, me
Ah'm Rid
Ah shout ma name
Ah'll no be overlookit
Or mistooken
No me
Ah'm in your face
Ah'm Rid
No like thon icy-lippit Blue
Or sapsy Broon
Ah've got attitude
Ah'm up for it
Ah'm hot
Move ower'n let the talent through
Ah'm Rid

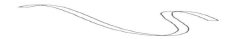

Blue

Hing loose
That's what ah dae
Ah'm Blue
Ah'm cool
Ah'll no be hassled
Wi the likes
O in-yer-face Rid
No me
Ah'm cool
Ah've got style
Ah dinnae need
Tae shout ma name
Ah'm weel kent
Ah tak the weight aff ma feet
An chill
Ah'm Blue
Ah'm cool

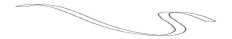

Black

Ah'm the boss o the gang
Ah'm the king o the castle
Ah've been aroond
Whit ah say, goes
Wha'll staund against me?
Naebody
Ah've got the strength
Ah've got the power
Ah can make a'thin dark
Respect me
Ah'm Black

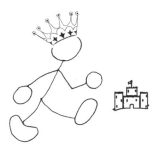

Orange

Ah like tae show aff
Sing a song
Hae a pairty
Bring the Irn Bru
Dance the Hokey Cokey
Let ma hair doon
Forget aboot the morra
Come on, enjoy yersel
Sook me
Ah'm Orange

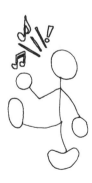

Pink

Touch ma pale
Candy floss saftness
Hug me
Whisper gigglin secrets
as ah aim to please
But dinnae get
Ower familiar
Cos aneath the surface
Ah can be as hard
As chewed bubblegum
Spat on the street
Yet ah'm a guid pal
Tae Mental-Rid an Show-Aff-Purple
Ah let them tak the lead
But behind the scenes
Ah pull the strings
Me, Pink - the wan who aims
To please

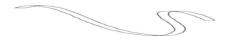

Grey

Some colours call me
A wattered doon black
As dreich as rain
Black's lackey
But ah'm a peacemaker
Ah try tae keep a'body happy
Cos ah can see baith sides
O the spectrum
It's hard gaun sometimes
An ah get fair scunnered wi it a'
But ah dae ma best
Ah really dae
Ah'm Grey
But sometimes
Ah'd raither be White

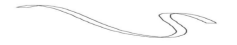

Yellow

Ah'm cheery
Ah'm freenly
Ah'm a guid neebur
Ah'll mix wi onybody
Ah'm a ray o sunshine
A splash o me
Taks the blues awa
Hae a go
Dinnae haud back
Spread me aboot
Ah'm Yellow

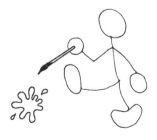

Fawn

Can ye see me
At a'?
Ah blend in
Ye can tak me onywhere
Ah fit in fine
Ah'm no pushy
Efter you is whit ah say
But ah get there
Ah'd mak a guid detective
Or a spy
Ah'd turn up the collar o ma coat
Slip in an oot
And naebody wid ken ah'm there
That's whit ah like
It's a quiet life
When ye're Fawn

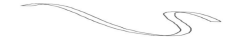

Fawn's Rap

Ah'm the colour o a biscuit
Ah'm the colour o a wa
If ah staund behind a lamppost
Ye'll no see ma face at a'

Whaurever ye may go
Whaurever ye may be
Ah'll see you

        But ye'll no see me

When ye're playin tig wi tigers
When ye're stripey as can be
Ah'll see you

        But ye'll no see me

When ye're slidin wi the penguins
When ye're slippy as can be
Ah'll see you

        But ye'll no see me

When ye're nibblin wi the squirrels
When ye're nuts as nuts can be
Ah'll see you

But ye'll no see me

Whaurever ye may go
Whaurever ye may be
Ah'll see you

But ye'll no see me

When ye're playin tig wi tigers
When ye're slidin wi the penguins
When ye're nibblin wi the squirrels
Whaurever ye may be
Ah'll see you

But ye'll no see me

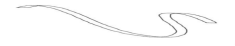

The Purple Bear

Ma sister's got a purple bear
Ah love it so ah dae
So sometimes when she isnae
there
Ah tak her bear away

Ah like tae rub its purple fur
An squeeze its wee black nose
But when ah hear her comin
Back tae its place it goes

Wan day ah took a notion
Tae gie the bear a baff
But when ah cam tae dry it
Its purple had washed aff

It turned intae a wee broon bear
So whit was ah tae dae?
Ah heard ma sister comin in
So she was on her way

Ah got ma maw's sunglesses
An pit them on its nose
Ah dressed it in the babby's vest
Tae gie it summer clothes

An when ma sister saw it
Ah said afore ah ran
Yer bear's been on its holidays
See, whit a lovely tan

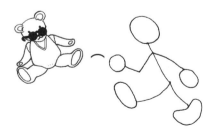

At The Disco

Rid goes tae the disco
Tae shake it a' aboot

See me?
Ah'm a mover
Ah'm a groover
Ah'm a disco babe
Says Rid

Silver appears
An strikes a pose

Are ye dancin?
Says Silver

Are ye askin?
Says Rid

Ah'm askin
Says Silver

Then ah'm dancin
Says Rid

Haund in haund
Rid an Silver
Birl aroond the flair
Haein a ball

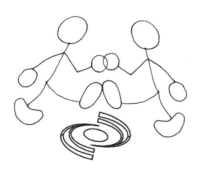

Summer Dreams

Ah'm slippin intae the waarm blue
watter
Lying oan ma back
Ma een shut
Ah could be a seal
Haein a dook
Afore sunbathin on the rocks
Ah could be a giant monster
Livin in the deep below
Ah could be a diver
Findin golden treasure
In a Spanish galleon
Ah open ma een
There's green in the watter
An wee sparkly bits whaur the sun
hits it
An whaur the green an blue meet
There's a colour that's baith o
them
Turquoise
The colour o the waarm sea
An ma summer dreams

The Colour O Happiness

(To the tune of I'm H-A-P-P-Y)

Ah'm Y-E-L-L-O
Ah'm Y-E-L-L-O
Ah feel ah am, ah hope ah am
Ah'm Y-E-L-L-O
Whit, speired Orange, happened
To the W?
It fell aff an goat lost
So it's nowt tae dae wi the fact
That ye canny spell?
Nah
Ye're a daft gowk, dae ye ken
that?
Aye, but it disnae bother me cos
Ah'm Y-E-L-L-O
Ah'm Y-E-L-L-O
Ah feel ah am, ah hope ah am
Ah'm Y-E-L-L-O

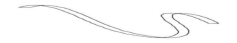

Paintbox Story

Splash me on yer paper
Dip yer brush in
Show me aff
In a' ma glory
Gie me leaves tae dress
Jumpy frogs an humpy caterpillars
Paint wi nature
Say ma name
Green

Let me drip ontae yer page
Like strawberry jam
Drap thick dauds o me
Spread me aboot
So a'body can see me
Paint wi life
Say ma name
Rid

Wash me ower yer page
Wi a big brush
Golden licht
Liftin up yer hert
Makin ye smile
Paint wi sunshine
Say ma name
Yellow

Stretch me across oceans
Fill the sky wi me
Think big
See the sun rise an set in me
Paint wi abundance
Say ma name
Blue

A Scabby Tale

Ah fell aff ma skateboard
An banged ma knee ...

(*To the Tune of Ten in a Bed*)

It wis bleedin an rid
Then scabbed in broon
Turnin black at the edge
Giein me a wedge
Ah picked it ... ah picked it

Then a watery rid
Ran doon ma leg
Wi a yella goo
Which stuck like glue
Ah dabbed it ... ah dabbed it

It re-scabbed
Went broony an black
It looked real bad
And itched like mad
Ah left it ... ah left it

A fawn crust hung
And then fell aff
Noo ma skin's a' new
Wi a shiny pink hue
Ah'm fine noo ... ah'm fine noo
AH'M FINE NOO

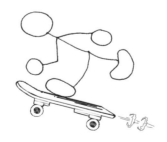

The Snaw Angel

Saft an silent it sneaked in
Smotherin the land an
Edgin oot the nicht
White
Polar-bear white
Snaw
Bright, crisp, even
Untouched by footprints
Until
Wan wee lass, happit-up
Against the cauld
Stepped oot in her pink wellies
An lifted her feet
Scrunch ... scrunch ... scrunch
Roon she went
Drawin oot her message in the
snaw

Until
She fell spread-eagled
Tae mak a snaw angel
That night the moon shone doon
On the snaw angel's
Footprints
The snaw angel in
Pink wellies
The snaw angel who
Had left a gift
Tae the night
Cos
In a' that bitter cauld whiteness
She had left ahent
Her hert

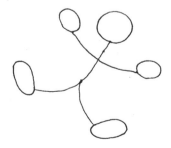

Cock-A-Hoopey Orange

(To the Tune of The Hokey Cokey)

Ye pit yer chuffed face on
Ye pit yer chest richt oot
Ye pit yer haunds up high
An ye grin fae ear tae ear
Ye go a cock-a-hoopey
An ye sparkle an fizz
Jist like orangeade

Go a cock-a-hoopey
Go a cock-a-hoopey
Go a cock-a-hoopey
Jist like orangeade

Ye pit yer chin richt up
Ye pit yer hips in a sway
Ye pit yer glad rags on
An ye go an hit the toon
Ye go a cock-a-hoopey
An ye sparkle an fizz
Jist like orangeade

Go a cock-a-hoopey
Go a cock-a-hoopey
Go a cock-a-hoopey
Jist like orangeade

Ye let yer fingers click
Ye let yer taes tap oot
Ye let yer hair hing doon
An ye dance the night awa
Ye go a cock-a-hoopey
An ye sparkle an fizz
Jist like orangeade

Go a cock-a-hoopey
Go a cock-a-hoopey
Go a cock-a-hoopey
Jist like orangeade

Wan Day (Green)

Wan day
The world will be green
A'body's mind will be green
Green thoughts will blossom
Whales will swim
in peace
Butterflies will flourish
An birds will sing
A green song
Nature an man will walk thegither
Wearin
Green

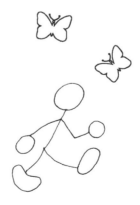

Wan Day (Blue)

Wan day
The world will be blue
There will be
nae mair fightin
Or fallin oot
Folk will tak the time
Tae listen an talk tae each other
How's it gaun neebur?
An ah'll gie ye a
haund wi that
Will be the in words
Folk will jist chill
An hing oot thegither
Aneath a sky's that
A' fu o blue

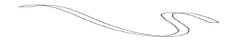

Wha's Haein A Great Time?

Wha is it
Kens a' the trees by name
Swims wi the dolphins
Shows the butterflies whaur the
flooers are
Has the time o its life?

Wha is it
Goes on holiday
Pits on the shades
Chills oot
Has a real cool time?

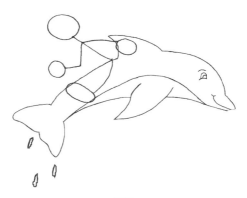

Wha is it
Eats a' the pies
Sings at the karaoke
Dances the hoochycoochy
Haes a real braw time?

Wha is it
Maks patterns on the winter
windaes
Pits crystal draps on the
chandeliers
Brightens up ony place
Has a brilliant time?

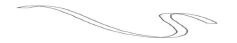

The Colour O Secret Fears

Ah hug the night
Gie folk a fright

Ah can be mean an bad
But sometimes sad

Ah'm the colour o secret fears
An sometimes ah'm the cause o
tears

Ah hear the screams
Fae weans wi scary dreams

And feel the poondin o a hert
O wan who wakes up wi a stert

Ah linger roon late-night bars
But ah'm the pal o the moon an
stars

Ah just hide
Ma safter side

An cosy it up just like a pup
Keepin wan safe till the sun
comes up

Ye see, ah like the light
The end o night

Black an white
We are alike

We need each ither
Like sister an brither

Opposites dae attract
But ah like the fact that ah am
black

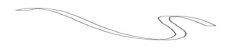

The Rainbow Rap

Comin oot ma fingers
Comin oot ma feet
Rainbow rhythm
Rainbow beat
In ma shooders
In ma croon
Someweys up
And someweys doon
Let yer taes oot
Fur a tap
Jivin tae the rainbow rap

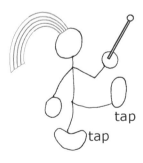

Comin oot ma fingers
Comin oot ma feet
Rainbow rhythm
Rainbow beat
Wi a toot
An wi a blaw
Wi a bang an crash anaw
Let the planet
Ken ye're there
Mak it dance
An ask fur mair

Let yer taes oot fur a tap
Jivin tae the rainbow rap

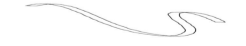

A Richt Stooshie

There wis a richt stooshie in the
world o colours
A'body wis arguin
And no getting on wi each ither
Until
A rumour began tae dae the roons
The world o colours wis aboot tae
change
It wis tae become monochrome
Black an white

The colours were feart
Awfy feart
They a' got thegither
Whit will we dae? they a' asked
Grey
Ye can start by makin up
An being pals again, Grey
answered
Mak the world a better place
Broon thocht aboot it an then
looked at Rid

Ah'm sorry ah said that ye were
that mental
That ye were a danger tae yersel
That's okay, replied Rid an ah
didnae mean it
When ah said ye were the colour o
Rotten teeth

Ye're no a wee snotter
said Pink to Green
Hauding Green's haund
An so a'body made an effort
To tak a' their bad words back
Even Black jined in
Cos wi'oot colours who wid
He hae tae boss aroond?
Grey smiled
Rumours come in handy
sometimes
Especially if ye start them
Yersel

Fadin Awa

Whit is it? asked Purple
It's a colour, said Grey,
But Ah'm no sure which colour
Blue thocht it could be
A green gaun wrang
Poor soul, put in Pink,
the colour's a' washed oot
It must be gey auld

The colour started to fade
Even mair
Whit's it sayin? asked Purple
Pink leaned in close
Bleach, Pink squeaked, the colour's
Been bleached

A shudder ran roon them a'
As they watched Colourless
Become fainter an fainter until
It completely disappeared

They a' bowed their heids

Bleached to death, said Grey,
Whit a way tae go
Aye, drawled Blue, gone to that
Rainbow in the sky

At that they a' looked upwards
An what they saw astoonded them
Ah guess it wis a rid, said Purple,
See, it's shoutin its name
An so it wis
As the sun began to set
Rid wis showin aff a' ower the sky

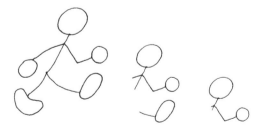

Walkin The Rainbow

The sun lit up the smirr o the rain
An then an arch o colours
appeared

A rainbow, whispered Pink
A' the colours gawped at White

Except Black - Black scowled

Aye, it wis a rainbow, said White
The colours a' held haunds
An danced a' ower the sky

Wis indigo and violet
Haudin hands? Purple asked
Aye, an rid an orange an yellow
An green an blue

Pink an Purple were fair chuffed
They did high-fives

Black scowled even harder

Ahm stappit fu o guidness
Said Green, ma colour
Wid hae tae be there

Ah'm the colour o talent
Anaw, Rid shouted

An orange an yellow,
We aye dance thegither,
pipped up Orange

Weel, drawled Blue, strummin
The guitar, Ah'd rather walk
Than dance the rainbow

Black wis ragin
Richt - Fawn, Grey an Broon
We're oot o' here, *noo*

Wait, shouted White
I havenae feenished

Aye ye have, growled Black

Just haud yer tongue an listen
Fawn blends in wi a' the colours
Makin them stronger

Broon, the rainbow bows its
Heid to touch the broon o earth

Grey, ye're in the smirr o the rain
Which brings us the rainbow

An Black, ye're special tae
Wi'oot you the moon and stars
Couldnae shine
A' the colours gawped at White
Including Black

An they a' thocht the same thing
That White wis rather special tae
In fact
White wis pure deid brilliant

44

Mingin Mawkit An Broon

Ah dae ken whit a'body's
Gangin up against me fur
Ah'm no tryin tae wipe
Oot a' the colours
No me
Ah cannae help bein
Broon
An doon tae earth
It's jist the way ah am
An it's no ma fault
That a' the colours got
A' clarted up in glaur
An cam back mawkit
An mingin
An a' broon
They're a sicht so they are
Come tae think o it
Some o them
Look almost as guid
As me

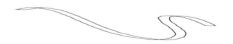

Colourful Thochts

Hae a guddle
In a puddle
Jump up an doon in it
Jist for badness
Enjoy yersel
Says Orange

Mak stairhead pieces
Spread them thick
Share them oot
wi yer pals
Be generous
Says Yellow

Climb a tree
Gie a cuddyback
Plant a seed
Says Green

Gang tae the disco
Strut yer stuff
Be bold
Says Rid

Aim high
Like the snaw on the mountains
Be your best
Says White

Staund up an be counted
Dinnae be feart
Dae yer ain thing
Says Black

Jine in
Or stey oot
Be prood o who ye are
Says Fawn

Stick yer tongue oot
An turn yer face up tae the rain
It maks for a guid day
Says Grey

Noo and again get yer
Haunds dirty
Revel in no being perfect
Says Broon

Gie yer pal a hug
Yer mam and dad a kiss
Embrace life
Says Pink

Be courageous but
Laugh wi and no at yer freens
Says Purple

Jist lie back
And dream dreams
Never lose them
Says Blue

Be colourful a' yer life

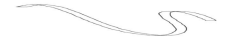

48

WINDFALL BOOKS

LILLIAN KING
2 RAILWAY COTTAGES
WESTCROFT WAY
KELTY KY4 0AT

Phone: 01383 831076
Fax: 01383 831076
lillian@king1288.fsnet.co.uk
www.windfallbooks.co.uk

Enclosed is a copy of the Book
for you to have a look at as you
have been working with Sheryl for
may years to say a few words about the
and the Book at the Launch. Look
forward to seeing you then.

Lillian

With Compliments

The Rainbow Story

Wance
A rainbow fell
Intae a puddle
An a' the folk that passed by
Wet an grumpy
Wi their umbrellas an shopping
bags
Saw it
An said
Naw
It cannae be
Wha ever saw a rainbow
In a puddle?
Then a wee boy cam
He saw the rainbow
An he fished it oot
An took it hame
An pit it in his hert

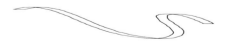

Glossary

ahent - behind
chuffed - very pleased
clarted – dirtied, muddied
cuddyback - a ride on someone's
back or shoulders
dauds – dabs
dreich - dreary
dook – swim
een – eyes
feart - afraid
freens - friends
glaur – mud, ooze or slime
gowk –fool
guddle - fish with the hands by
groping underwater
guddle - messy work
happit up – dressed up
mawkit – filthy
mingin – stinking
neebur – neighbour
scunnered – bored, disgusted,
fed up

smirr – fine rain, drizzle
speired - asked
stairheid - landing at the top of the
stairs
stairheid pieces - sandwiches
thrown out of tenement windows
to children waiting below
stappit fu – full up
stooshie- uproar
weans - children

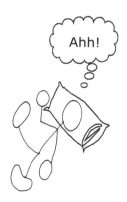

Poems by Elizabeth Cordiner

Imagine
Rid
Black
White
Green
Orange
Yellow
Fawn
Fawn's Rap
The Purple Bear
At The Disco
Summer Dreams
Paintbox Story
Wan Day(Green)
Wha's Haein A Great Time?
The Rainbow Rap
The Rainbow Story

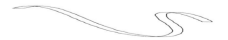

Poems by Jill Bennett

Blue
Broon
Purple
Pink
Grey
The Colour O Happiness
A Scabby Tale
The Snaw Angel
Cock-A-Hoopey Orange
Wan Day (Blue)
The Colour O Secret Fears
A Richt Stooshie
Fadin Awa
Walkin The Rainbow
Mingin Mawkit An Broon

Poems by Elizabeth Cordiner and Jill Bennett

Colourful Thochts

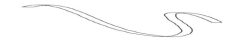